Coping with
Crohn's Disease

Manage Your Physical Symptoms and Overcome the Emotional Challenges

Amy B. Trachter, Psy.D., Ph.D.

New Harbinger Publications, Inc.

Publisher's Note

This publication is designed to provide accurate and authoritative information in regard to the subject matter covered. It is sold with the understanding that the publisher is not engaged in rendering psychological, financial, legal, or other professional services. If expert assistance or counseling is needed, the services of a competent professional should be sought.

Distributed in the U.S.A. by Publishers Group West; in Canada by Raincoast Books; in Great Britain by Airlift Book Company, Ltd.; in South Africa by Real Books, Ltd.; in Australia by Boobook; and in New Zealand by Tandem Press.

Copyright © 2001 by Amy B. Trachter
New Harbinger Publications, Inc.
5674 Shattuck Avenue
Oakland, CA 94609

Cover design © by Lightbourne Images
Edited by Kayla Sussell
Book design by Michele Waters

Library of Congress Catalog Card Number: 01-132290
ISBN 157224-265-5 Paperback

New Harbinger Publications' Web site address: www.newharbinger.com

03   02   01

10   9   8   7   6   5   4   3   2   1

First printing

This book is dedicated to the wonderful people who were my support system during the most difficult times of my life, thank you so much. May all patients who live with this disease be blessed with the opportunity to have people like those listed below in their lives: *Arlene and Michael, Muriel, Judy, Judy and Arthur, Adam, Sari and Matt, Alicia and Steven, Susan and Michael, Sheryl, David, Michelle, Joel and Adele, Brook, Lisa and Gary, Brooke and Marc, Joan and Cliff, Marcia and Saul, Beth and Jeff, Debbie and Todd, Eve and Mark, Mindy and Michael, Terry and Jerry, Tom and Rachel, Merle and Daryl, Trish, Debbie and Sue, Rick, Jeff, and Scott, Deborah and Steve, Mary, Diana, Marianne and Gerhart, Dr. David Lipkin, Dr. Henry Wodnecki, and especially, Dr. Charles M. Rosen.*

Contents

PART II
Emotional Challenges

Foreword

When the average person first learns that he or she has Crohn's disease, two questions are usually asked: They are "What is Crohn's disease?" and "What will my life be like now?" The brief answer to the first question is that Crohn's disease is a chronic gastrointestinal inflammatory disease that may affect any part of the digestive tract. The second question is a lot harder to answer because it is a disease that affects everyone differently.

The disease process can be somewhat mild, or it can be devastating. However, the diagnosis of a chronic medical condition can be overwhelming. It is even more so when the initial diagnosis is made for a very young person. Chronic illnesses can cause a great deal of stress in the patient's relationships with family and friends. Body image and self-esteem can be adversely affected.

This book addresses not only the emotional aspects of living with a chronic illness, but also the physical. Nutrition is a very important factor. The gastrointestinal tract may not respond as it did before the disease presented. A person with Crohn's disease must learn which foods to avoid, while having to learn all over again how to maintain a complete, healthy, and enjoyable diet.

Today, an overwhelming amount of information about Crohn's disease exists, but until now, a source that is both precise and concise has been lacking. Patients, families, and friends will find this book to be a great resource in navigating through the maze of information about Crohn's disease. Let us dispel the myths and work with information that will help us feed both the body and soul!

—Henry Wodnicki, M.D.
Mount Sinai Medical Center
4302 Alton Road, Suite 810
Miami Beach, FL 33140

Preface

Coping with Crohn's Disease developed from the needs of people who live their lives with Crohn's disease. As an individual who also lives with Crohn's disease, I have learned invaluable lessons that I do not believe I would have otherwise experienced. Writing this book was important to me from a personal perspective because it gave me the opportunity to share information with others that would have been helpful to me. During the periods of my life when I had active disease, I felt a range of emotions. However, through my own personal experiences as a medical patient, I gained a unique insight and empathy for the individuals whom I have been privileged to treat.

As an individual who is a psychologist, the majority of my clinical experiences have been with people who have medical illnesses. Throughout my professional endeavors, I have tried not only to understand the hardships that people encounter in life, but also the feelings surrounding those hardships. I genuinely cared for all the people whom I have treated. Additionally, the other physicians and psychologists with whom I have worked have been exceptionally compassionate and caring individuals, as well as excellent teachers.

At the beginning of undertaking this project, I was determined to write this book from my professional viewpoint. My professional experiences provided me with a solid background of composition skills; they also gave me clinical experiences from which to describe the case examples in this book. I have provided psychotherapy to people on both inpatient hospital units and outpatient clinics. While there were times that I believed my experiences as a patient were helpful to those I treated, I am sure there were times they were not. As all interactions with people are biased to some degree by who we are, I am certain that mine were, as well. However, I tried to do the best job that I could, given my life experiences.

The Preface was the last part of this book that I wrote. As I complete it, it is symbolic of the end of a chapter of my own life. My experience writing this book has reminded me of how far I've come from the ill younger woman I once was, and how my acceptance of this illness and my experiences surrounding it, have had a great impact on the person I am today, on the quality of my life, and the quality of my relationships with people. Although I may carry a diagnosis of Crohn's disease on my medical chart, I continue to pursue my life goals and am determined not to simply exist but to live.

As an author, I have written this book with the intent of providing people with helpful information, motivation to develop the inner strength and courage that living with a chronic illness can require, and hope for the future. I shall remember this wonderful learning experience with fondness, gratitude, and appreciation for the treasures that life's opportunities have provided, most especially those relating to my disease. When I think of all the extraordinary individuals, who have been, continue to be, and become a part of my life as a result of Crohn's disease, I am overwhelmed with gratitude.

The information in this book is based on the combination of both my personal and professional experiences. It contains words that are often spoken among patients, but not always placed on paper. It is my hope that as you read this book, you will not only find helpful information, but also recognize the rainbow after the storm, which may, at times, be hard to see. *Coping with Crohn's Disease* was written with the purpose of making life easier for people who have Crohn's disease, that is, the normal day-to-day activities, situations, and interactions with others.

Although this book provides basic medical information, it is designed to be used as a tool to aid the activities of daily life, as well as to promote a healthy lifestyle, despite the disease. The writing is clear, easy to understand, and does not require a medical background. Medical terminology has been kept to the barest minimum and a glossary of terms is provided in an appendix at the back of the book. Each chapter may be read independently of one another. Although identifying information has been significantly altered, the case illustrations presented throughout the chapters are all based on real people who live with Crohn's disease.

Acknowledgments

To New Harbinger Publications, with special gratitude to Jueli Gastwirth, Acquisitions Editor, Heather Garnos, Senior Editor, and especially Kayla Sussell, Copy Editor, for guiding me through the process of writing this book. Thank you to Dr. Morton Katz, for without his support and suggestion, this project would not have taken place. Thank you to the Crohn's and Colitis Foundation of America for giving me the opportunity to work with amazing people and providing me with quality friendships. Thank you to Dr. Kiron Das for allowing me the privilege of learning from a great teacher. Thank you Dr. Neil Stollman for his unconditional support and time. Thanks to Patricia Silk for her patience, reading, and feedback.

A special heartfelt thanks, sincere appreciation, and much gratitude to Dr. Arvey I. Rogers, who has supported, encouraged, and facilitated my professional endeavors, who has been generous with his time, bestowed his wisdom, and who was the catalyst for my involvement in all of the aforementioned activities.

Thank you to Dr. Stephen Weiss for the guidance, advice, and time that you kindly and graciously provided.

Thank you to Dr. Christopher C. Corrie for your confidence, wit, and grace.

With appreciation and gratitude, many thanks to Dr. Henry Wodnicki, for graciously and kindly writing the foreword of this book.

Thank you to my parents, Michael and Arlene, for bringing me into this wonderful world, and to Dr. Henry Wodnicki, for keeping me here.

PART I

Physical Considerations

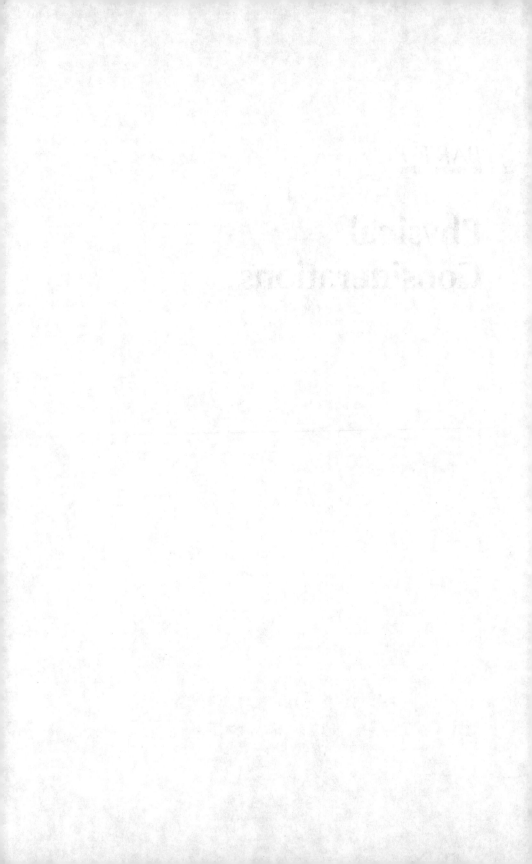

Chapter 1

Crohn's Disease: What Does It Really Mean?

If you are reading this book, the chances are that you have, think you have, or know someone who has Crohn's disease. Most people who have heard about Crohn's disease find out about it because they have it or know someone who has it. If you are reading this book, you have a head start on helping yourself. Why? Because information is helpful, and the more informed you are about your disease, the better able you are to help yourself.

Definition

So what exactly is Crohn's disease? It is a gastrointestinal inflammatory disease that may affect any part of the digestive tract from the mouth to the anus. It can affect your esophagus, stomach, intestines, and/or rectum. This doesn't mean that it will affect all of these organs in your body, just that it might. For the majority of people, Crohn's disease typically affects the small and/or large intestine, or colon. "Colon" and "large intestine" are synonymous, and the terms will be used interchangeably throughout this book.

What Causes Crohn's Disease?

The cause of Crohn's disease is unknown. However, it is thought that the disease results from a deficiency in the immune system, such that the body attacks itself in the digestive tract, most often in the intestine. The full lining of the intestinal wall is affected, which means that every layer of the diseased intestine is affected, making it difficult for food to pass through, or to be digested properly.

Because Crohn's disease may affect any part of your digestive tract, it is important for you to be aware of those parts of your digestive system in which the disease is located. Understanding where the disease is located in your body will also help you to understand why you are taking certain types of medications.

Crohn's disease may affect one area of your digestive system at one point in your life, and another part of your digestive system at another time. For example, at the time of your diagnosis, you could have the disease in your small intestine, control it with medication, and feel fine for years. Many years later, Crohn's disease could become active again, but be located in your colon as opposed to your small intestine.

No one knows why Crohn's disease affects different parts of the digestive tract at different times. Crohn's disease, and its symptoms, may wax and wane throughout the course of your life. You may feel sick only once in your lifetime, and never have symptoms again. Conversely, you may feel ill off and on for years, depending on the disease activity in your body.

For example, a woman who was diagnosed with Crohn's disease at the age of forty-five had disease activity located near the ileum, in her small intestine. It was well controlled with medications prescribed by her physician. The disease went into remission, and didn't trouble her until eleven years later, when the disease became active in her body once again. She knew the disease had become active because of abdominal cramping and increased frequency of diarrhea. When the disease returned, it was still located in her small intestine, but in a different area of the bowel, illustrating that Crohn's disease can remit in one area and become active again in another. Her physician prescribed medication for her and she subsequently felt better.

It is important to remember that your disease is as individual as you are. No two people have exactly the same Crohn's disease, or exactly the same symptoms. Although it is a chronic illness without a cure (at the moment), it is, typically, not a life-threatening disease. Don't make judgments about your disease based on what you hear about other people's experiences—make judgments about your disease based on your own experiences. As you continue reading, this advice will become clearer to you.

Descriptions of Crohn's Disease

Crohn's disease, because it can affect any part of the digestive system, is identified based on where the disease is located in your body. Consequently, terms commonly used to describe Crohn's disease reflect *where* the disease is in your body. For example, *Crohn's colitis, small bowel Crohn's disease, ileocecal Crohn's*, and *perianal Crohn's* are typical labels, or categories, of the disease that you may hear from your physician. These labels for Crohn's disease do not mean that there are different types of Crohn's disease, as there are for different types of hepatitis, each with different causes and treatments. Crohn's disease is located in different parts of the body, but functions the same way regardless of where the illness is located, similar to cancer. The labels make it easier for professionals to communicate with one another.

The next section provides a brief description of some of the most common terms used to describe Crohn's disease. However, there are some terms that require clarification before the labels for Crohn's disease can be discussed. The definition of *colitis*, for instance, is inflammation of the colon, or large intestine. Sometimes there is confusion between the term colitis and *ulcerative colitis*.

Colitis or Ulcerative Colitis?

There are people who have *ulcerative colitis*, which is another type of inflammatory bowel disease. Although the two diseases (ulcerative colitis and Crohn's disease) are comparable in that the physiological symptoms of each include frequent bathroom use, abdominal pain, dehydration, and lethargy, there are pathophysiological (the study of how normal physiological processes are altered by disease) differences between the two. Crohn's disease affects the full thickness of the bowel wall, whereas ulcerative colitis affects only the inner lining of the wall of the intestine.

Ulcerative colitis affects *only* the colon, but, as you now know, Crohn's disease can affect any location in the digestive tract. Also, ulcerative colitis tends to be continuous, in that the disease tends to be located in the same place over time, whereas Crohn's disease is patchy, or tends to affect different areas of the bowel over time. Crohn's disease cannot be cured by surgery; ulcerative colitis may be surgically removed. Some people who say they have "colitis" may be referring to ulcerative colitis. However, they may also be referring to irritable bowel syndrome, which is different from both ulcerative colitis and Crohn's disease, and is another term that requires clarification.

Irritable Bowel Syndrome

Irritable bowel syndrome (IBS), like ulcerative colitis and Crohn's disease, also causes frequent bathroom use, abdominal pain, and cramping, but people with irritable bowel syndrome do *not* necessarily have inflammatory bowel disease (IBD). Those who have irritable bowel syndrome do *not* have any permanent damage to their intestines, or any part of their digestive system. Their intestines become sore in a manner that may cause diarrhea and cramping, but their symptoms do not usually require the medical and/or surgical interventions commonly used with people who have inflammatory bowel disease (Crohn's disease and ulcerative colitis). Now that you understand the differences between the types of inflammatory bowel disease and irritable bowel syndrome, the different names used to describe Crohn's disease will be a little easier to understand.

Crohn's Colitis

Crohn's colitis does not mean that you have both Crohn's disease and colitis; it means that your Crohn's disease is restricted to your colon, or large intestine. Any part of the colon, or your entire colon, may be involved. Typically, in Crohn's colitis the rectum is not affected.

Ileocecal Crohn's Disease

Ileocecal Crohn's disease means there is Crohn's disease in the terminal *ileum* and in the *cecum* just like it sounds.

Small Bowel Crohn's Disease

In *small bowel Crohn's disease*, Crohn's is usually restricted to the small bowel, and the terminal ileum may or may not be involved.

The symptoms of Crohn's colitis, ileocecal Crohn's disease, and small bowel Crohn's disease are all similar to one another. You will not be able to tell where your Crohn's disease is located exactly, unless you ask your doctor. The way to ascertain precisely where the disease is located in your body is through tests given to you by your physician.

Perineal Crohn's Disease

Perineal Crohn's disease refers to disease activity in the rectal or *perianal* area, which may appear as fissures (cuts), fistulas (see Appendix A: Glossary), and/or local inflammation. The perineum includes the anal and genital areas and their surrounding tissues. Approximately 25 percent of those with Crohn's disease experience difficulties with the disease in this part of the body (Janowitz 1994). Crohn's disease may appear in the area around the perineum, when the disease is active in the rectum, or large intestine. It may appear as redness, swelling, or inflammation around your rectal area. You may see fissures, or cuts, around your anus. Perineal complications include both abscesses and fistulas, which drain pus and/or bowel contents onto the skin, and/or perforate (create openings) into the vagina or scrotum.

Perianal fistulas are external tracts that may form from one area of the rectum to another. External, of course, means outer; tracts are abnormal tubelike passages. Thus, an "external tract" is a tubelike passage on the inside of your body that leads to an opening on the outside of your body.

These types of fistulas may form as a result of an abscess, which you can both see and feel. An *abscess* is an internal collection of pus, which may feel to you as if you are sitting on a "black and blue" bruise. Consequently, abscesses can be quite painful, unless they drain spontaneously, or are drained by a doctor. In Crohn's disease, an abscess ultimately may develop into a fistula. Remember, this *may* happen; that doesn't mean it *will* happen.

Perianal fistulas form tracts that drain fluid and pus from the opening of an area of the rectum, which usually closes with medical treatment. Crohn's disease can also cause slow-to-heal ulcerations, and new tissue growths around the anal area, called *skin tags*, which are often mistaken for hemorrhoids.

The Epidemiology of Crohn's Disease

Although you may think that Crohn's disease is uncommon, in fact, there are an estimated one million people in the United States with inflammatory bowel disease (Crohn's and Colitis Foundation of America 2000). This figure is likely to be an underestimation of the prevalence of Crohn's disease due to underreported cases, the delay in diagnosis, and the fact that most people are not hospitalized for their disease at the time of their diagnoses (Sandler 1994). Approximately 30,000 new cases of IBD are admitted to United States hospitals each year, with the incidence at 4.3 Crohn's disease cases and fifteen ulcerative colitis cases per 100,000 people (Sandler 1994).

Crohn's disease has its peak onset in adolescence and early adulthood. Inflammatory bowel disease is more common among whites as opposed to non-whites and Jewish people versus non-Jewish people (Alic 2000; Andres and Friedmann 1999; Monk, Medeloff, Siegel, and Lilienfeld 1970; Sandler 1994). According to Andres and Friedmann (1999), there are no gender differences among those with ulcerative colitis; the male to female ratio for those with Crohn's disease is 1:1.8. Crohn's disease is also more prevalent in people from Scandinavian countries, Great Britain, and North America (Sandler 1994).

The Role of Genetics

Although it is thought that there is a genetic component to Crohn's disease, it is unclear as to whether you will pass it on to your children. For example, there are some with Crohn's disease who have a history of the disease in their family. For these people, there is a greater chance of passing it along to their children. However, there are many people who have Crohn's disease and no one else in either their immediate or extended family has it; thus making genetic transmission less likely. No one knows conclusively whether you will pass the disease on to your children or not; there just hasn't been enough research in the area of genetic transmission of Crohn's disease to say with certainty.

As recently as May 2001, however, researchers were able to identify a gene that increases the risk of developing Crohn's disease. According to a press release by the chairperson of the CCFA National Scientific Advisory Committee, Charles Elson, M.D., on May 21, 2001, a gene known as Nod2 mutates such that it increases the likelihood of developing Crohn's disease. The Nod2 gene is a gene that is associated with the immune system, but exactly how the mutated gene increases the risk of Crohn's disease is still unclear.

According to researchers, having one mutated Nod2 gene doubles your chances of developing Crohn's and two mutated genes increase the risk fifteen to twenty times. A study conducted in Europe independently of the United States found the same results. The United States research study was funded partly by CCFA and conducted at both the University of Michigan and the University of Chicago.

Now that you have a greater understanding of what Crohn's disease is, the remainder of Part 1 of this book will discuss the physical considerations of the disease, including medical and surgical treatments, as well as your relationship with medical professionals. The rest of this chapter discusses both the physical and psychological reactions that you may experience.

The Physical Symptoms of Crohn's Disease

As the various symptoms and manifestations of Crohn's disease are described below, keep in mind that only some, and not all, may apply to you. If a symptom does not apply to you, do not become concerned. It does not mean that you eventually *will* have all the symptoms that are described. Remember, everyone's disease is different; what happens to one individual with Crohn's does not always happen to *all* individuals with Crohn's.

There are a variety of symptoms commonly experienced by people with Crohn's disease. Frequent diarrhea is the most common symptom. Sometimes, though, people experience severe constipation as a manifestation of the disease; constipation will occur if a segment of the intestine is blocked, such that food cannot travel through it.

However, your intestine does not necessarily have to be blocked for you to experience constipation as a symptom of Crohn's disease. You may see blood in your stool, or in the toilet. You may have cuts, or *fissures*, around your rectal area due to the frequency of going to the bathroom. You may experience *tenesmus*, which is the feeling of urgency that tells you "I need a toilet." You may also experience abdominal pain. Abdominal pain may accompany defecation, or it may simply occur periodically without warning throughout the day. You may find that you can eat much more than you usually do, and still lose weight. This may mean that the food you eat is not being adequately digested, and you should see your physician.

You may find that there are specific times of the day when your symptoms occur. For instance, after you wake up, you may spend most of the morning in the bathroom. Or you may spend most of your evening in the bathroom after having eaten all of your meals for the day. If you talk to different people with the disease, you will find that, typically, most people have a specific time of day that is especially troublesome with regard to spending more time on the toilet. It is up to you to discern what that time of day is for you. Notice when you feel the urge to go, and note to yourself when you use the bathroom most often. This will assist you in making the appropriate adjustments in your lifestyle, as well as provide you with relevant information to share with your doctor.

Why is this type of information important to share with your doctor? Although this will be covered in more detail in the next chapter, suffice to say that physicians need as much *accurate* information from you about your disease as possible. Accurate information helps your doctors figure out what is the most appropriate form of treatment for you, and it assists them in providing you with the best care possible.

Extra-Intestinal Manifestations

There are some symptoms of Crohn's disease that are referred to as "extra-intestinal manifestations." This is because some people experience symptoms that are indicative of Crohn's disease, but do not involve the digestive tract. These include, but are not limited to, skin rashes or pyoderma gangrenosm, erethyma nodosm (red lumps on your legs), joint pain, eye infections or uveitis, and chancre sores.

Extra-intestinal manifestations are not that common. Some people experience them as a consequence of disease activity, some as a consequence of medications, and still others have comorbid conditions.

When you have a comorbid condition, it means that you have more than one condition or illness that is active at the same time. If you have arthritis, for example, it will be hard for you to know whether the joint pain you feel is due to the arthritis or to Crohn's disease. This is another reason for telling your physician about *all* of your symptoms. Let your doctor decide what the cause of your symptoms is; it is your doctor's job. However, it is your job to know what your symptoms are, and to tell your doctor about them. Physical symptoms of Crohn's disease may or may not be difficult for you to tolerate. One thing is certain, however; you do have feelings and emotional reactions to your disease—whether you like having the disease or not.

Psychological Reactions to Your Diagnosis

As you read this book, you might consider keeping a separate journal of your thoughts and feelings. You may find that some of the thoughts and feelings described in this book are familiar to you. A journal will allow you to identify your thoughts and feelings easily, those that are in agreement with what you read, and those that are not. Also, a journal helps you when you feel physically well, as it can serve as a concrete reminder of how much you've learned along the way.

All of the physical symptoms described above are unpleasant. As a result, you may have a variety of emotional responses and reactions to your symptoms. Everyone feels something about their symptoms—it is a natural human reaction. Who wouldn't have an emotional response to frequent pain and/or diarrhea? The rest of this chapter discusses the range of emotional responses you may have to your symptoms and provides suggestions on how to handle those reactions. Furthermore, the second half of this book deals entirely with the emotional challenges of living with Crohn's disease.

People have a wide variety of different reactions to finding out that they have Crohn's disease. Most often, their initial reactions are disbelief and shock. After all, how can defecation, a universal human behavior, be so bad? How can having to use the toilet frequently mean you have a disease? And what exactly does having Crohn's disease mean to you?

Well, it means different things to different people at different times, depending on their disease activity. Unfortunately, what it means to everyone who has it, especially initially, is that you have a chronic illness that has no cure. You're stuck with it for the rest of your life. Unless a cure is discovered in your lifetime, you have a chronic illness, and that is a fact that will not change. This fact often leads to a range of emotions, including shock and disbelief, denial, fear, anger, depression, worry, concern, and frustration.

Denial

Denial is a frequent, common reaction to initial diagnosis. Shock is a part of denial. Perhaps you don't know what "Crohn's disease" means and you ask your doctor to tell you all that he or she knows. It is not uncommon to hear the words "Crohn's disease" for the very first time at the time of your diagnosis. You may walk away from the doctor's office taken aback, confused, sad, angry, or some variant of all of these. These emotions are all natural, normal reactions to experiencing a loss.

Yes, if your diagnosis is that you have Crohn's disease, you've experienced a loss. A loss of the "healthy" person you were, up to the minute before your physician said, "I know what's wrong with you. You've got Crohn's disease." However, just because you have a chronic illness doesn't mean that you are not capable of living a healthy life. On the contrary, you *are* capable of living a healthy life, you just have to adjust and make accommodations in your life in a manner that nurtures the *part of you* with the illness.

How to Handle Denial

Inherent in denial is the fact that you do not want to handle or deal with your disease. Denial is not uncommon; however, sometimes it can get you into trouble. If you do not have an active disease, or your disease is in remission, denial may work very well for you. After all, if your disease isn't bothering you, you don't have to deal with it.

But the lapse into denial also can be a problem for those who have inactive disease. For example, if you are the kind of person who stops taking your medication when you feel better, and do not discuss it with your doctor first, you might be causing yourself some harm. Although medications and their side effects and consequences are discussed in greater detail in later chapters, it is important to remember that the lapse into denial can cause you greater difficulties if you do not monitor yourself with your physician. This means that even when you're feeling well and your disease is not active, you should see a physician periodically (every two to three years).

If you do have symptoms of the disease and you are in denial, you may cause yourself greater difficulties over time. For instance, if you are having symptoms and try to ignore them, that may work for you for a while. But, if your symptoms are not treated, they will, most likely, worsen with time and cause you even more difficulty. If you are unsure as to whether you're in denial, ask yourself the following questions:

1. Am I having symptoms and not telling my doctor?

2. Am I having symptoms and not telling anyone about them?

3. Am I reading this book and thinking that I don't feel any of these emotions: disbelief, denial, fear, anger, depression, worry, concern, and frustration?

If your answer is yes to any of the questions, the chances are good that you are experiencing, at the very least, some denial. If you are experiencing symptoms of disease, and you haven't called your doctor yet, please, put the book down now, and call for an appointment. As you continue to read, you will see how important communicating with your physician becomes. Besides, the faster your symptoms are treated, the faster you will feel better.

Anger

Anger is another emotion many people experience when they find out they have Crohn's disease. You may be angry because there is no cure. You may be angry because you have to take medication. You may be angry because your life has been disrupted by the need to use the bathroom frequently. Sometimes, you're even angry at those around you for not understanding how going to the bathroom so often can be so disruptive. You may be angry and frustrated, and rightfully so.

Yet, there is no one person to blame—no one to whom you can say, "Hey, it's your fault this happened to me!" So you are left with all this anger, and nowhere to direct it. Consequently, you might find yourself agitated or frustrated over some unrelated event that typically wouldn't bother you at all. Although anger is an understandable and natural reaction to learning that you have Crohn's disease, how you express your anger may either help or hinder your disease.

How to Handle Anger

Anger is an extremely powerful emotion. It can energize you in a way that most emotions do not. Think of all the energy you use when you are angry. Now think of what you could do with that energy if it were directed in a way that was beneficial to you. You can choose to handle your anger in a way that is helpful to you, or not, but first you must identify what anger means to you. For instance, ask yourself the following questions and, on a separate sheet of paper, write your answers:

1. How do I know I'm angry? How do I react when I am angry?

2. Can other people tell when I am angry? How do they know?

3. Do I think anger is a "positive" emotion or a "negative" emotion? Why or why not?

4. Is my behavior different when I'm angry? How so?

Answering these questions will assist you in identifying how you express anger. It is also helpful for you to become familiar with the types of situations and events that cause you to become angry. Do you think your anger is always justifiable? Or only in certain situations? When do you become angry? Has expressing anger been difficult for you? If so, how? By answering these questions, you will increase your awareness of what triggers your anger. Learning about what makes you angry will help you to express your anger in more effective ways.

Your body reacts physically to anger. This very strong emotion may cause blood pressure, blood flow, heart rate, and muscle tension to increase (Antoni, Schneiderman, and Ironson 2000). The next time you get angry, observe how your body feels. It is likely that you will notice the tension in your muscles readily. Identifying ways to manage your anger effectively will help you not just with the anger you may feel about your illness, but in other situations, as well.

Sometimes people exercise to help manage their anger reactions. Physical activity might be working out in the gym, swimming, walking, jogging, or whatever physical exercise brings you enjoyment. For some people, however, physical exercise is very difficult because they are simply too sick and/or too tired to engage in such activities. For these people, handling anger through physical activity becomes more difficult, but not impossible. Physical activity, for instance, might involve rearranging your closet, polishing your silverware, or waxing your car.

If even those kinds of physical activity are too difficult, try writing down your feelings in a journal. It may seem as if anger cannot be expressed adequately in this manner. However, when you're really angry, there are a number of chemical and hormonal changes that take place due to the "fight-or-flight" physiological responses activated by anger. Many people find that writing journal entries about how they feel—while they are feeling those adrenaline surges—actually helps them to express their anger more accurately and effectively.

Effectively communicating your feelings of anger may also be helpful to you. When you can express yourself in a way that demonstrates how you are feeling, without yelling or becoming emotionally upset, you are more likely to be heard. However you choose to handle your anger, try not to hold it inside. Holding on to your anger internally will not help you feel better emotionally. Besides, if you hold your anger in, it is likely to affect your gut, and who wants that?

Ways to Express Anger

1. Discuss your feelings of anger in an effective, assertive manner with someone you trust.

2. Do physical exercise of any type (walking, jogging, biking, swimming, etc.).

3. Write about how you are feeling in a journal.

4. Rearrange closets, drawers, cabinets, shelves, etc.

5. Do arts and crafts activities (sewing, knitting, drawing, etc.).

6. Engage in household activities (painting, wallpapering, gardening, polishing silverware).

Depression

Depression is another common reaction that people with Crohn's disease experience at some point after their initial diagnosis. At first, the loss of one's robust physical health is very sad; there's no way around it. You can mourn the loss, however, and continue on with your life. You will, at times, have to adapt to accommodate the disease activity in your body, whether you want to or not. That fact can be depressing.

It is easy to become depressed when you are experiencing chronic pain. Or when you can't eat the food you like, are tired all the time, and are having difficulty sleeping. Depression, like anger, denial, and anxiety, is a normal human response to a chronic illness and/or chronic symptoms. Depression makes it easier to allow yourself to stay near a bathroom, where you are safe from accidents, than to go out into the world and have to explain to others that you have chronic diarrhea. After all, when you are depressed, it may be easier to isolate yourself rather than explain why diarrhea is hampering your lifestyle.

It is precisely at those times, however, that you must try to find the inner strength to go beyond the day-to-day frustrations and see the bigger picture. *Be patient. Your symptoms will not last forever.* In time, your symptoms will remit, and you will feel better. It is when you are feeling physically tired and ill, that patience becomes a virtue.

If you want to have a "pity party" for yourself, fine, go ahead. You are entitled to take some time off and say, "I'm sick of being sick." But give yourself a time limit; too often people become so involved with their symptoms, they become their diseases. Too much pity isn't healthy for you either. You run the risk of allowing the disease to *become your life*, instead of *just a part of it*.

Certainly, initially, having a "pity party" is a normal reaction. A pity party takes place when you say to yourself, "Why me? Why do I have to have this disease?" Or you might decide to have a pity party when your symptoms become active, and you say to yourself, "Why is this happening now? Why can't I just be healthy and feel good like everyone else?" Although this can be a healthy release for pent-up emotions, if your pity party lasts longer than a day or two, it can lead to your feeling increasingly sad and depressed. So monitor yourself. If you are asking yourself these kinds of self-pitying questions, please realize that most people with Crohn's disease ask themselves these questions at one time or another.

However, it is important not to become so involved with the whys that you become entrenched in the disease process. Don't allow the disease to become your entire life. Ultimately, you are in control of your thoughts, your feelings, and your behaviors. Allow yourself the time to feel sorry for yourself without becoming destructive to your psyche. Help yourself by consciously stopping the pity party after a limited amount of time. For some people, this period might be a single day, for others it might be a week, or even two. But set a time limit for yourself, and stick to it. Whatever time frame you allow for yourself, bear in mind the longer your pity party lasts, the longer it will take for you to become actively involved in helping to ease your disease, both physically and psychologically.

How to Handle Depression

Although you may feel sad that you have been diagnosed with a chronic illness, and rightfully so, there are things you can do to help yourself. First, don't think about your disease and your symptoms *all* the time. Involve yourself in activities that make you feel better, whether they are with others or by yourself. Going to the movies, reading a book, gardening, or engaging in arts and crafts activities can be done alone or with others. They are not too strenuous and all can be done near a bathroom.

If you really want to help yourself, the best thing you can do when you are feeling down is to get away from your disease for a while. Do anything that takes your mind off it. Even if it is for only a few minutes at a time. Don't allow the disease to take over your life!

There are many ways to handle depression and sadness. Although there is a list of suggested activities below, accessing additional resources and information also will be helpful. Obtaining information about your disease will assist you in feeling some sense of mastery over it, which will, hopefully, provide you with a greater sense of control over the disease process taking place in your body. Social support is also very helpful in overcoming depression (see chapter 9). See also chapter 6 for a discussion of the interactions between your emotions and your disease, and how your attitude can help you prevent sadness and depression.

Ways to Handle Depression

1. Involve yourself in activities that take your mind off the disease (arts and crafts, movies, reading, talking on the phone, etc.).

2. Seek psychotherapy with a clinician who is familiar with Crohn's disease.

3. Obtain social support (from family, friends, or wherever you get support). See chapter 9.

4. Write down all of your thoughts and feelings about Crohn's disease (see the last section of this chapter).

5. Be good to yourself. Do relaxing and pleasant activities that make you feel good (take warm baths, listen to or play music, watch a comedy).

Anxiety and Fear

Anxiety is one of the most common emotions that Crohn's disease generates. Initially, lack of information regarding the disease promotes anxiety, because you may not understand what the diagnosis will mean for you. The more information you have, the less anxiety you may experience, because you will know what to expect. However, the disease itself also creates anxiety. You never know when you're going to need a bathroom. You never know when the "urge to go" is going to hit you. Thus, your life revolves around where the bathrooms are "just in case" you need one.

Fear plays a role in anxiety related to Crohn's disease, as well. In any situation, fear of the unknown may produce anxiety. There are many questions about Crohn's disease that remain unanswered. Unanswered questions provoke frustration in patients and doctors alike. It is difficult to handle a disease properly when you have only limited information, which is why having as much information about your disease as is possible will be helpful to you in decreasing your anxieties and fears.

It is natural to feel anxiety, fear, and worry as a result of frequent bathroom use, chronic pain, and all the other symptoms of Crohn's disease. Emotions like these may engulf you at any time. You may find, however, that there are particular situations that provoke these feelings. It is important for you to identify those situations that provoke the most anxiety, so that you will know how to take action to decrease your fear and anxiety.

Robert's Fear

For example, consider Robert's story. Robert was a thirty-three-year-old man, with Crohn's disease, who worked as an administrative assistant in a big law firm. For years, his desk was fairly close to the company's rest rooms. When he was promoted, his workspace was relocated to a much larger area, a room with a window. However, the new workspace was also quite far from the bathrooms. No one in his firm knew of his illness, and he began to experience increasing amounts of anxiety because of his worry about "having an accident" and not being able to get to the bathroom in time.

Robert's anxiety increased to such an extent that he finally broke down and explained his situation to his supervisor. Without any further ado, his supervisor promptly relocated Robert's desk once again, so as to decrease his anxiety and the level of distraction his worry had created for him, and to accommodate his disease.

That's just one example of several different types of fears that will be discussed in detail later in the book. For now, it is important to remember that there are things that you can do to decrease your anxieties and fears. Because the cause of Crohn's disease is unknown, there isn't much that anyone can do to prevent getting the disease. However, there are ways you can help yourself once you have been diagnosed. The rest of this chapter (and the rest of the book) focuses on how to live with your disease.

Identifying Your Reactions to the Diagnosis

Before you can handle your reaction to your diagnosis, you must identify your reactions: what it is that you are feeling and thinking. Remember, there are no right or wrong ways to handle Crohn's disease. Whatever works for you is the right way. But if you don't know how to deal with it at all, it is important to identify your reactions, so that you can learn how to deal with it.

Knowing what your reactions are likely to be will help you to improve your communications with your physician, family, and friends. It will assist you in *helping yourself* to feel better, and it will make it easier for you to target what kind of help you may need from your loved ones. Identifying your reactions will give you a greater understanding of yourself, and ease your adjustment to your illness.

Step One: Identify Feelings and Thoughts

Feelings aren't right or wrong, they just are. Think about what you felt when you found out you had Crohn's. What was going through your mind? What did you feel? Sadness, fear, anger, uncertainty? What was it like for you? What did you say to yourself? Did you tell other people? Why or why not? What were you thinking about yourself? What were you thinking about the disease?

Step Two: Write About How You Felt and What You Thought

Make a list. Write down everything you thought and felt when you were first diagnosed. Decide whether your thoughts and feelings matched up with one another. Did you know that every thought you have is related to some type of feeling? It's true. For instance, the thought "I can't believe this is happening" might be related to the feeling "numb," or to the feeling of "surprise." The thought, "This can't be true, I'll get a second opinion" might be related to anger or denial.

Write about how you feel about your body now that you know you have Crohn's. You really want to get in touch with what you think about yourself as it relates to your disease. Writing about your thoughts and feelings provides you with examples of the inner dialogue that only you hear. Writing about your feelings often can reveal thoughts you didn't even know you were thinking. This exercise will assist you later on when you reach the second part of this book because you will be more aware of your own thoughts and feelings. Here is an example of what your list might look like:

Feelings	Thoughts	Behavior
Anger	"I hate this disease."	Yelling, shouting, impatient Harsh tone of voice
Depression	"Why did this happen to me?" "I don't want to have this disease."	Crying, quiet, isolation
Fear	"What's going to happen now?" "Will this ever go away?" "What am I going to do?"	Isolation, going to the bathroom even when you do not need to use the toilet
Anxiety	"I don't know where the bathroom is in this place. Where is it?" "Am I going to have an accident?"	Isolation, decreased socialization, shaking, increased heart rate

Step Three: Identify Behaviors Related to Your Thoughts and Feelings

Once you have your list of thoughts and feelings that you had in response to your diagnosis of Crohn's disease, relate those thoughts and feelings to your behavior after your diagnosis. Did you tell people? If so, who? If not, why not? Are you more aware of which bathrooms you use? Do you use the handicapped bathroom stall in public rest rooms now? Why or why not? Are you more aware of where the bathrooms are in public places? Are you more conscientious about when and where you use the toilet? Do you plan your days around when you go to the bathroom? How do such behaviors tie in to your thoughts and feelings? Add these behaviors next to your list of thoughts and feelings. Make note of how they are related, and what that relationship tells you about yourself in the context of your disease. Be honest with yourself. It is much harder for others to help you if you can't identify what your needs are.

Step Four: Keep Your List Handy

Your list of feelings, thoughts, and behaviors will help you in your interactions with others. Specifically, it will help you to communicate your specific needs to your physician and to the significant people in your life. It will also help you evaluate your reaction to other people as well as their reactions to you. Keeping the list easily accessible will sharpen your own awareness of your thoughts and feelings and how they influence your behaviors. The list can act as a reminder for you when you are feeling badly, or need to obtain some help for yourself.

Another way you could choose to use the list is to rid yourself symbolically of those thoughts and feelings that you don't want to continue having. For example, suppose you are particularly anxious about attending a work-related meeting. Write down all the negative thoughts and feelings you have about the meeting, and then throw out the list. Crinkle it up and toss it in the garbage; rip it to shreds; place it in a paper shredder. Get rid of those negative thoughts and feelings.

Accept the Fact That You Have Crohn's Disease

Once you have identified how you feel, think, and behave, you will be able to act in ways that will decrease your negative emotions and increase your positive ones. You've chosen to read this book to help yourself. To truly help yourself, you have to accept yourself for who you are, including the Crohn's disease, which is a part of who you are.

You may choose to separate yourself from the disease, and split yourself into two: you with the disease and you without the disease—but if you truly want to help yourself, that's not the best idea. Although having a disease for life seems harsh right now, hopefully, there will come a time when you will be so used to having Crohn's, that it will seem as natural to you as the color of your eyes or hair. This book was written to help you do just that.

Chapter 2

Relationships with Medical Professionals

The relationships you develop with the medical professionals who treat your disease is integral to your treatment. Throughout the course of your lifetime, you will see many medical professionals to assist you with your health problems. You will interact with doctors, nurses, social workers, and, depending on where you receive your treatment, psychologists and nutritionists, as well. The relationships you develop will be helpful not only to the treatment of your disease, but also to your overall feeling of well-being. Why? Because these are the people who will be your greatest source of support and security when you are feeling physically ill and vulnerable. This chapter explains why your relationships with medical professionals are important to the treatment of your disease, and discusses how to maximize those relationships, so that you do, indeed, receive the best treatment possible.

The Importance of Your Relationship with Your Doctor

Everyone sees a doctor at one time or another in their lives. As an individual with a chronic illness, specifically Crohn's disease, your relationship with medical professionals, particularly your doctor, is especially significant. Your physicians are the people who are going to support you the most, as they are the people who are the most knowledgeable about your illness. They provide you with the greatest support because they are the people who treat your disease.

Your relationship with your doctor is important for several reasons. First, because you have an illness that does not have a cure, a physician should monitor you periodically throughout your lifetime, regardless of whether the disease is active or not. Second, you want to be able to trust your doctor without any reservations. Your doctor is, after all, the person who is your greatest supporter throughout the treatment of your disease.

Ideally, you want to have a collaborative relationship with your physician. A collaborative relationship involves mutual trust, respect, and honesty between two (or more) people. You want to be able to be completely honest with your doctor and feel comfortable discussing your disease, your symptoms, and the treatments that have been prescribed and/or recommended to you. You want to *form an alliance with your physician against the disease*. Moreover, you want to feel sufficiently comfortable with your physician to discuss topics that may be indirectly related to your health, such as difficulties with work and/or partner relationships.

A collaborative relationship is especially critical for people with Crohn's disease. Why? Because the nature of Crohn's disease varies so much from individual to individual, doctors need as much accurate information as possible from *you*, the patient. For example, Crohn's disease is not a disease like diabetes. As a rule, a person with diabetes feels ill, and his or her blood sugar is tested. Based on the results of the blood sugar levels, the exact dosage of insulin can be calculated that will make that person feel better. Crohn's disease doesn't work that way. A doctor cannot calculate *exactly* how much of a certain medication will work for your disease activity, unless you communicate your symptoms as honestly and openly as possible. *Disease activity* refers to the symptoms of disease that you are experiencing. Later sections of this chapter focus on how and what to communicate to your physician.

Why Your Relationships with Other Medical Professionals Are Important

Your relationships with other medical professionals are also valuable to the treatment of your disease because they will facilitate a good working relationship with your physician. Your physician's coworkers, such as nurses and administrative staff, may be of assistance to you. These are the people who function as liaisons with your physician, and often communicate how you are feeling to the doctor. They schedule your appointments and fit you into your already busy doctor's schedule. For instance, if you call your physician's office in acute distress, with abdominal pain, cramping, and increased diarrhea, typically, it will be the nurse with whom you will speak, until the doctor is available. It will be a member of the doctor's support staff who gives you an appointment.

It also will be beneficial for you to develop collaborative relationships with the nurses. The nurses, like you, follow the doctor's instructions. Nurses assist physicians with medical procedures, such as the preparation for testing and blood work. For those people who are in the hospital, nurses administer the medications prescribed by the physician. Nurses often act as the contact person between you and your physician, so, clearly, it will be helpful for you to develop good rapport with them. When the medical professionals your physician deals with daily collaborate with each other, their cooperation can be very helpful in the treatment of your disease. However, before you can communicate to your physician you have to find one.

Finding a Physician

Most people find out they have Crohn's disease from a gastroenterologist. A gastroenterologist is a doctor who specializes in diseases of the digestive system. As a rule, people go to their primary doctor's office to report stomach problems. If the primary doctor suspects that Crohn's disease is the culprit, the primary doctor usually will refer the patient to a gastroenterologist, to ascertain that, in fact,

Crohn's disease is present. There are occasions, however, when the primary care physician does the necessary testing and does not refer the patient to a gastroenterologist.

A gastroenterologist is a physician who has received specialized training specifically in the diseases of the digestive tract. You may or may not like and trust the gastroenterologist your physician refers you to for diagnostic purposes. If that is the case, follow the suggestions outlined in the next section, "How to Find a Physician," to find a gastroenterologist whom you do like.

The gastroenterologist is usually the physician whom you will see when you are feeling ill and having problems with your disease. Because Crohn's disease is yours for life (sorry about that), entering into a trusting, honest doctor-patient relationship from the start will be extremely helpful to you. Note that many gastroenterologists want their patients to check in with them periodically (every couple of years), even when they are feeling well and not experiencing any symptoms at all.

How to Find a Physician

There are several ways to find a physician. First, you can see the gastroenterologist referred to you by your doctor. You also can ask your doctor to give you more than one gastroenterologist's name. Another good way to find a gastroenterologist is to ask a patient like yourself for a doctor's name. Other people who have Crohn's disease are really good sources for finding a physician because they will have had the same procedures performed on them (i.e., colonoscopy, flexible sigmoidoscopy).

If you don't know anyone else with Crohn's disease, call up the local chapter of the Crohn's and Colitis Foundation of America (CCFA) and explain your situation (see Appendix B). Give them your phone number and ask them if they would contact a patient for you, and ask that patient to call you, so that you can speak directly to him or her. The Crohn's and Colitis Foundation of America will provide you with the names of doctors who are members of their local organization.

You may also want to inquire whether the gastroenterologist your primary care physician referred you to is a member of the organization. This recommendation doesn't mean that there are not plenty of excellent gastroenterologists who are not members of CCFA. There are. It just means that those physicians who are members are aware of the organization that supports patients in the Crohn's and colitis community. See chapter 9 for a detailed description of CCFA and how it can be of assistance to you.

Communicating with Your Physician

Communicating well with your doctors is always important to your physical well-being. However, good communication is especially salient for you, as a person with Crohn's disease. There are two major reasons for this. The first is the fact that the symptoms of Crohn's disease vary from person to person. The second is that everyone's disease is not always located in the same place in the digestive tract. Your doctor needs as much information about your symptoms as possible, so that she/he can prescribe the most appropriate treatment.

For example, Jon a forty-two-year-old man, newly diagnosed with Crohn's disease, was prescribed a particular amount of prednisone based on the symptoms he had told his doctor he was experiencing. He said that he was going to the bathroom four times a day, and experiencing abdominal cramping both prior to and during defecation. Indeed, Jon was having diarrhea four times a day. However, he failed to mention that he was also being awakened from sleep three to four times a night to go to the bathroom, as well. After hearing that, the doctor altered the dosage of the medication that had been prescribed originally. Eight times in a *twenty-four-hour period* is different from four times in a twenty-four-hour period. The different types of medical treatments and their effects are discussed in detail in chapter 3.

What Should You Tell Your Physician?

There are several things to tell to your physician. First, you want to describe the symptoms of your disease. This includes how many times you go to bathroom in a twenty-four-hour period. As in the example above, sometimes people forget to mention that they get up in the middle of the night to go to the bathroom. Your doctor needs this information to assess the disease activity in your body accurately. Furthermore, if you aren't going to the bathroom at night, you need to say so. You also will want to tell your doctor about any abdominal cramping, muscle or joint pain, vomiting, and/or any other physical symptoms that you have recently experienced.

Stress

You also need to inform your physician about any unusual or "stressful" situations currently taking place in your life. Stress does *not* cause Crohn's disease; however, it may exacerbate your symptoms, or make them occur more frequently. For example, let's say your disease is active, but controlled with medication. Perhaps you are going to the bathroom twice a day. Now, let's say that, recently, you were told by your boss that a project you thought you had a month to complete is now due in less than a week. After hearing this information, you may find yourself going to the bathroom more frequently and experiencing additional abdominal pain for several days. Again, this is not to say that stressors like this *will* increase your symptoms, only that they might. In any case, it is important to let your doctor know what is happening in your body, and to reveal anything in your life that might indirectly affect your disease. See chapter 6 for a discussion that deals specifically with stress and its relationship to your disease.

What Should You Ask Your Physician?

You may ask your physician any questions that you have regarding your disease. It is essential that you understand how the disease affects your body. If someone told you that you had cancer, you would ask where it was, right? The same holds true for Crohn's disease. Ask your physician where the disease is located. This will help you to understand why certain medications might be prescribed for you. It will give you a greater understanding of your own body, and help you adjust to the "new" you. You also may want to ask how much of your digestive system, or intestine, is affected. Again, if you were told you had cancer of the pancreas, you would want to know how much of your pancreas was affected. The same holds true for Crohn's disease. Ask your physician how much of your intestine is affected. The more information you have about the disease, the better able you will be to understand it, integrate it, and help yourself adhere to a healthier lifestyle.

If you don't understand something that your doctor explains to you, tell that to him/her. Ask for another explanation, or ask her/him to direct you to a source that can explain it so that you will understand what is happening to your body. It is always good to ask your doctor where to obtain current, relevant information about your disease. This is a question that can help you for several reasons. First, it assists you in obtaining valuable information about Crohn's disease. Second, it demonstrates your interest in learning about the disease to your physician, which may improve communication between the two of you. And, finally, it is a protective question, in that it checks whether your doctor is, in fact, aware of recent developments, and can direct you to the newest (or relatively new) information about treatments for the disease.

You may also want to ask about the medications you are taking and what possible side effects you may encounter. It is always useful to inquire about possible side effects so that if you should experience one (or some), you do not become alarmed. For example, if you take prednisone for an extended period of time, you might notice some swelling on the back of your neck. This is commonly referred to as a "buffalo hump," and it is just one of many *possible* side effects that might occur. It disappears when the prednisone is stopped, so don't freak out if this has occurred. (Also, don't freak out if this hasn't occurred, because it may not happen to you.) See chapter 3 for a discussion of medications and their side effects.

Honesty Is Always the Best Policy

Of course, you are going to be honest and open about your symptoms. As previously stated, you do yourself a disservice if you do not communicate your symptoms in an open and honest manner. If you are taking medications and you start to feel better, you may not feel like taking all of the medications that were prescribed for you. It is *usually* in your best interest to follow the directions of your physician. However, if you are not going to listen, have the courtesy and respect for the person treating you to say, "Doctor, I just wanted you to know, I stopped taking my Asacol." At least in this way, the doctor knows what is going on in your body *without the medication*. Otherwise, your physician might think that your disease is functioning differently from what is really happening. Honest communication about adherence to your medical regimen also helps to maintain the trust you've established with your physician.

Questions to Ask Your Physician

1. Where is the disease in my body?

2. How much of my digestive system/intestine is affected?

3. What are the usually prescribed treatments for my disease?

4. Why have you chosen drug "A" over other medications? How does it work? When will it begin to take effect?

5. What are the side effects of drug "A"? How likely is it that I will experience such side effects?

6. Where can I find out more about my disease? What books can I read?

7. Should I be on a special diet or taking nutritional supplements of any kind?

8. Is there anything else I can do to help myself feel better?

Other Matters to Discuss with Your Physician

Generally speaking, for most people, life isn't easy. Life with Crohn's disease just makes life slightly more complicated. It is important for you to share information with your physicians that affects the quality of your life. For instance, certain life events are stressful for *everyone*, regardless of whether they have Crohn's disease or not. Stressful life events may or may not affect your illness in that your symptoms may increase during stressful times. A new job or new relationship, weddings, births, moving, divorce, and the death of loved ones are life events that are stressful for everyone. However, stress *does not cause* Crohn's disease. If events like these are taking place in your life, tell your doctor. Not because these events *will* make you sicker but because they *might* make your symptoms increase. Besides, if you have a good relationship with your physician, you will most likely want her/him to know about such life events anyway.

It is also beneficial to talk to your doctor about events outside of your disease activity, such as when you experience difficulties in certain environments. For instance, if you are worried about the stability of your job and/or your relationship, or if you have any issue that is causing you to be particularly anxious or concerned, share this information with your doctor. Physicians need your help. They can't know what is going on with you if you don't tell them.

Compromising Is Helpful

For example, a twenty-seven-year-old woman, Alice, went to see her gastroenterologist because her Crohn's disease was acting up. She was going to the bathroom more frequently, and was having "accidents" at work. Her disease was located in her colon and rectum (Crohn's colitis). Alice hadn't been taking any medication for a while, because her disease had been inactive for some time. Her physician said that he was going to prescribe Rowasa suppositories to treat her disease. Alice responded, "You can prescribe them to me, but I don't do suppositories."

After some discussion, they reached a compromise. Alice's doctor agreed not to prescribe suppositories, but would prescribe Asacol, an oral medication, with the stipulation that Alice would return to the office in two weeks to be reevaluated. Alice agreed to take the Asacol *exactly* as prescribed for the two-week period. If, by the time of her next visit, her symptoms didn't improve, she agreed to take the suppositories until her disease activity diminished. This is a good illustration of how open, honest communication between physician and patient can facilitate medical treatment that is acceptable to both parties involved. It demonstrates how a doctor and patient can work together in a collaborative relationship to treat the disease in a manner tolerable to *both* of them.

Confirming Your Physician's Opinion

There may be times when confirming your physician's opinion is something that you wish to do just for your own peace of mind. Doctors aren't perfect; they are human beings just like everyone else. If you have any doubts about what your doctor has recommended to you, always ask her/him about it. If you are not satisfied with the answers you receive, there is no reason not to seek another doctor's opinion. However, it is always best to communicate with your physician first, before contacting additional or adjunctive services. You may feel somewhat awkward seeking another opinion. But if you have a good relationship with your doctor and communicate your desire and your concern, it should not be a problem. Besides, if your doctor is confident that what is being advised for you is the appropriate course of action, he/she will be likely to encourage another doctor's opinion. There are, however, some circumstances in which you will want a second opinion, regardless of your relationship with your doctor.

Confirming a Diagnosis

It is not always necessary to confirm a diagnosis. However, sometimes people find it helpful to confirm their diagnosis by a second doctor. You may decide to confirm your diagnosis simply because you need to hear it from another person to make it real to you. Regardless of your reason, if you are going to get a second opinion to verify the fact that you have Crohn's disease, you want to seek a physician who is known for his/her diagnostic acumen.

Most often, the physicians associated with medical schools have the most up-to-date information, techniques, medical equipment, and procedures. You want your second opinion to come from an "expert," or from someone affiliated with an "expert." Any physician associated with a medical school would be a good person to ask. If you don't live near a medical school, it might be worth a trip simply for your peace of mind. If that won't work for you, call the American College of Gastroenterology physician referral service. They will provide you with names of doctors in your area. For those people with Internet access, you can obtain the number of the American College of Gastroenterology at http://www.acg.gi.org/ (or see Appendix B for their phone number and/or address).

Confirming Treatment Recommendations

Recommendations for certain types of treatments may also be the impetus for seeking another physician's viewpoint. There will be times when your physician will say things to you that you will neither like nor want to hear. Again, there is nothing wrong with seeking another perspective. This is your disease, your body, and you are the one taking the medications. So, if your physician recommends a treatment that you don't think you can tolerate, and you cannot arrive at a mutual compromise, it may be the time to seek another viewpoint.

When Do You Know It Is Time for Another Opinion?

It is time for another opinion when you, the patient, do not feel comfortable with what your doctor is saying to you. Although doctors know the most about your disease, you know the most about yourself. You know which medications you will take as prescribed, and you also know what you won't do. You need to tell this to your doctor first, and if you get a response that makes you feel uncomfortable, or unsure of yourself, you need to tell this to your doctor, as well. Sometimes people are afraid to disagree or to confront their doctor with a question or the difficulties they may be experiencing. But if you don't tell your doctor what you are feeling and thinking, your silence will only make it more difficult for your doctor to treat you. Moreover, it will not facilitate a trusting and honest collaborative relationship. Remember, you are the patient, and obtaining more than one opinion can never hurt the treatment of your disease.

If surgery is recommended, that is the time when it is especially useful to obtain another opinion. Surgery is a big deal. If your doctor is recommending that you have surgery, you want to be sure that you have explored all other medical treatments available to you. Furthermore, when surgical treatment is involved, it is very reasonable to obtain a second opinion. See chapter 4 for discussion of specific surgical treatments and advice on how to obtain a surgeon who will be right for you.

There are other times it might be helpful to seek another doctor's opinion. For instance, if you are following your doctor's advice, and not feeling any better over a long period of time, seeking another physician's opinion for consultation purposes might be helpful to your treatment. "A long period of time" means that, if you are following your doctor's directions *and* you are not feeling any better after several months, *and* your doctor says to you, "This is the best I can do for you," get another opinion.

Sometimes, you may have such a good relationship with your doctor that you don't question anything he/she says, even though what's happening in your body doesn't seem right. It is wonderful to have a good relationship with your physician, but if you're not feeling better, it may be time to seek some additional and/or adjunct assistance.

Trust Your Physician and Your Body

Consider Alexander's story. Alexander was a twenty-three-year-old man with Crohn's disease who was placed on 6 Mercaptopurine (6-MP), or Purinethol (discussed in detail in chapter 3), due to severely active disease. Alexander was having his blood drawn weekly to monitor his immune system. After two months, he felt much better. His disease went into remission, and he was able to stop taking all the other medications he had been ingesting except the 6-MP. Due to the nature of 6-MP, Alexander was still receiving regular blood tests, although not on a weekly basis. During his third month of taking the medication, he began vomiting and feeling nauseous on occasion. He called his physician and told her of his symptoms. She told him not to worry; vomiting is sometimes a symptom of Crohn's disease. Alexander, trusting his physician completely, went about his daily routine and continued to go for his regular blood tests.

Six weeks later, Alexander's nausea and vomiting had increased; he figured the medication wasn't working as well as he wished. One day, his boss told him that she had noticed he was jaundiced and vomiting. She asked him whether he had hepatitis. Alexander denied having hepatitis, but he told her that, in fact, he did have Crohn's disease. His boss suggested that he should contact his doctor again and to mention that the whites of his eyes had turned yellow. When his physician heard that the whites of Alexander's eyes had turned yellow, she told him to come in for an examination immediately. Tests revealed that, indeed, he had drug-induced hepatitis (an uncommon side effect of the 6-MP). Unfortunately for Alexander, although the 6-MP resulted in remission of his disease, his liver couldn't tolerate the drug (the intolerance to the drug manifested in the form of hepatitis). When he stopped taking the 6-MP, the hepatitis disappeared.

Alexander's situation illustrates how you can do great harm to yourself when you place too much trust in your doctor. It also demonstrates that you should trust your body. Had Alexander been more assertive with his physician about his physical symptoms, the hepatitis might have been detected earlier. If you do not feel better with the treatment prescribed by your doctor, and you communicate your lack of improvement to her/him, and he/she does nothing, that would be a reasonable time to seek the opinion of another doctor as a consultant to help in your treatment.

If you know that you usually don't experience a certain symptom from Crohn's disease, such as vomiting, the chances are good that the symptom is due to something else going on in your body. Trust yourself. If you think there is something unusual happening inside of you, it is worth communicating your thoughts to your physician and having yourself examined.

What If the Second Opinion Disagrees with Your Physician's First Opinion?

If the second opinion disagrees with your doctor's first opinion, the situation can get a little sticky, but you do have options available to you. If you are looking for a second opinion, typically, it is because you are not feeling well and want to feel better quickly. Thus, you should weigh the two opinions of the doctors that you have, and speak with *other patients* who have followed the recommendations of *each* of the two physicians with whom you have consulted. Ask both physicians if they have any patients who are following the regimen that was recommended for you, and ask if they have patients who might be willing to speak to you. See what other patients say about the treatment that's being considered *and* the doctor who is prescribing it. In this way, you can make an informed decision about the medical regimen (and physician) that you feel would be most appropriate for you.

Ultimately, you are in charge of your body. You are the person who lives with the decisions that you and the medical professionals treating you make. That is why you must be able to recognize those decisions you can live with from those you can't. Taking care of yourself means (1) knowing what you can live with, and (2) enlisting the aid of medical professionals who can help you to live your life in the healthiest manner possible.

Chapter 3

A Medical Problem: How Is It Treated?

Chapters 1 and 2 discussed what Crohn's disease is and who is likely to provide you with treatment. Now, the actual treatment of your disease requires consideration. How will you be treated? How (and when) will you actually start to feel better? What will you have to do? Will you have to take medication forever? The answers to these questions are found in the remainder of the first half of this book. Both medical and surgical treatments for Crohn's disease, as well as how to handle the daily trials and tribulations of living with the physical symptoms of Crohn's, are addressed.

As you read, please keep in mind that these are treatment options some patients *may* experience, and not necessarily treatment options that *you* will experience. Throughout your reading try to remember that although living with a medical illness isn't always easy, it isn't the end of the world either.

Readjusting Your Life

Accommodating your life to a chronic illness often means using medications to help you feel better. Taking medication isn't something that most people enjoy doing, or wish to do. But if medication will help you to feel better, why not take it? Sometimes, taking a look at the bigger picture helps you keep it all in perspective, and helps you to overcome the physical symptoms and emotional demands that you may experience as a consequence of having a disease.

So, what does living with a chronic illness, Crohn's disease in particular, really mean? Well, it means you may have to take medications, and that you may have to have surgery one day. It means you may have to watch what types of food you eat, and it means you may always want to know where the nearest bathroom is located. It means you may experience, both physically and emotionally, painful situations that you'd rather not have to deal with at all. You will need to figure out how to integrate this disease into your life in a way that works for you.

Figuring out how to incorporate this disease into your life takes time, and it is a process that is different for everyone. Crohn's disease isn't the end of the world. Lots of people live long, productive lives with Crohn's disease. You can do anything anyone else can do. Try to remember that fact during the times you are feeling down and blue. Although it can be both frustrating and difficult to be happy when you are feeling physically ill, try to remember that your symptoms eventually will pass, and you will feel better in time. The rest of this chapter is focused on the medications that might be prescribed for you, and how they might affect you, so that you will have a greater understanding of the medical options available to you.

Remember that every patient is different and every doctor is different. Doctors may or may not prescribe certain drugs. There is not only one way to treat Crohn's disease, there are many treatment options available. Thus, you may hear of many different types of medications only some of which your doctor uses and prescribes for you. That's okay. It is likely that some medications are more appropriate for your disease than others.

Medications and Their Effects

As was stated in chapter 1, the cause of Crohn's disease is unknown. For that reason there is no medication you can take that will "cure" your disease. There are, however, many medications available to help you control your symptoms and feel better on a daily basis. Consequently, the goal of medication therapy is to control your symptoms and decrease or eliminate the inflammation in your digestive tract. Medication helps to ease abdominal pain, stops diarrhea, and treats inflammation.

Some people are lucky and, hopefully, you are one of them. Sometimes people need to take medication for only a brief period of time and their symptoms go away for a long time. When your symptoms cease and you feel well, your disease is considered to be in *remission*. A remission period can last from several weeks to many years. Some people experience long periods of remission and don't use medications during this time. Other people require maintenance medication so that their disease remains in remission. *Maintenance medication* can be any type of medication your doctor wants you to take even when you are feeling well, in order to keep you asymptomatic, that is, free of symptoms. The importance of maintenance medication is discussed later in this chapter.

Nonspecific Medications

Disease activity can be controlled with medications that are not specifically targeted for Crohn's disease. For instance, abdominal pain and diarrhea are symptoms that are not unique to Crohn's disease. Many people have these symptoms and do not have Crohn's. So, there are over-the-counter medications that help to control these symptoms. Antidiarrheal agents and pain medications are typically used as short-term treatment and/or as supplemental treatment to disease-specific drugs.

Antidiarrheal Agents and Pain Medications

Many antidiarrheal agents that are helpful to Crohn's patients can be purchased in your local drug store. Food poisoning, viruses, and/or flus can cause diarrhea, independent of a Crohn's disease diagnosis. Lomotil and Ioperamide (Imodium) are effective in reducing diarrhea whether it is caused by Crohn's disease or not. In these agents, the medication treats the symptoms without treating the underlying, or primary, cause of the symptoms (i.e., Crohn's disease).

Pain medications are another type of nonspecific medication that might be prescribed to you to for abdominal pain. Dicyclomine

(Bentyl) is a good example of a medication that is sometimes prescribed for pain. Tylenol with Codeine, Percocet, Darvocet, Merperidine, and Demerol are other pain medications sometimes used with Crohn's disease patients. However, these pain medications can be addicting, in that, over time, the body develops a tolerance to them. A *tolerance* to a drug means that after a period of time, usually two to four weeks, the effect of the drug decreases, and the patient needs more of it to work. Therefore, if you can find a way to control your pain without using pain medications, it is best for your body. (See chapter 5 for ways to manage and control your pain without the use of pain medications.)

Antibiotics

Antibiotics are another class of nonspecific medications that can be used to control your symptoms. The type of antibiotic that is prescribed has much to do with the type of symptoms you are experiencing, as well as your drug or medication history. For instance, many people are allergic to certain antibiotics; so, naturally, these antibiotics would not be prescribed. Antibiotics such as ampicillin, cephalosporin (Keflex), and/or tetracycline seem to improve Crohn's disease symptoms. Ciprofloxacin (Cipro) is another antibiotic used to treat Crohn's disease. Cipro is prescribed to people with Crohn's because it fights infection. However, medications such as these are considered nonspecific because they were not specifically developed to treat Crohn's disease.

Of all the antibiotics, metronidazole (Flagyl), appears to have specific effectiveness in Crohn's disease. Specifically, it appears to be of assistance in closing perineal fistulas and improving the overall symptoms of Crohn's disease. It is absorbed rapidly by the intestine and finds its way into all of the body fluids, appearing within minutes on the mucous membranes of the mouth, intestinal tract, and genitourinary system. The side effects of Flagyl include a metallic taste in the mouth, nausea, decreased appetite, sore throat, or "furry" tongue. A "furry" tongue is the result of bacterial changes in the mouth. Dark urine is a common side effect, as are headaches, skin rashes, and hives.

Antibiotics are frequently prescribed when people with Crohn's disease are in the hospital, usually in addition to the other medications they are t aking. Antibiotics are prescribed when people are hospitalized to help fight infection when the immune system has been compromised. The antibiotics function in a manner that provides some additional protection when the immune system is especially vulnerable. This is not always the case, but such prophylactic treatment is not unusual.

Many people respond well to such nonspecific medications, in conjunction with a well-balanced diet. Because people with Crohn's disease have frequent diarrhea, nutrition and diet are also quite important. Nutritional deficiency can occur as a consequence of frequent diarrhea. (See chapter 10 for a discussion on nutrition and eating patterns.)

Medications to Avoid

You should not use any medications to which you experience an allergic reaction. While this may seem obvious, it is important to remember those drugs that cause you to have adverse reactions. A particular medication may make your Crohn's disease symptoms feel better, but if it causes you to have other problems, it may not be worth taking. In a situation like this, a consultation with your physician is warranted.

You may also want to reconsider using drugs that contain aspirin or ibuprofen. The chemical agents in aspirin can increase bleeding and cause inflammation. If you have a headache, drugs without aspirin (e.g., Tylenol) may be the best way to help your headache. However, this is definitely a question for your physician. Everyone's experience with Crohn's disease and its medical treatment is unique. Many people take other medications for other reasons, as well. You need to ask your physician if there are any over-the-counter drugs that you should not take, to ensure and protect your health. You also need to tell your physician if there are other medications you are currently taking for other medical and/or psychological conditions, including any nutritional supplements, such as vitamins and minerals. Information like this provides your physician with a comprehensive idea of what's happening in your body.

Disease-Specific Medications

There are several disease-specific medications that are currently available to people with Crohn's disease. As you speak with other people who live with Crohn's disease, you will find that medical regimens differ among individuals. That's because, as previously stated, everyone's disease is different. Don't become concerned if the medications you are using are different from those used by someone else you know with Crohn's. It is likely that the reason for differing medications is due to different disease locations and/or activity.

Also, some physicians prefer certain types of medications over others, which is another reason why you and your friend or acquaintance with Crohn's may have different medical regimens. Again, do not become concerned. The best way to resolve a question about a type of medication you are taking is simply to ask your physician. Your friend isn't going to understand *your* disease as well as your doctor does. So accept what your friend says about *his/her medication*, and remember that it applies to *his or her disease*, not to yours.

The rest of this chapter describes the medications currently available to people with Crohn's disease and the possible side effects of these medications. It also discusses the process of taking medications, and how this process may affect you. You may be more familiar with some of these medications than others; but that's okay. Some of these medications may be inappropriate for you. This discussion is simply to provide you with the available options.

Corticosteroids (Prednisone and Methylprednisolone)

Corticosteroids are used to treat Crohn's disease patients because of their anti-inflammatory nature and their ability to suppress acute attacks of Crohn's disease. They were one of the first drugs used to treat Crohn's, as they have been around for years. For example, when Crohn's disease was called regional enteritis, corticosteroids were used for treatment. In fact, for a long time, corticosteroids were the only drugs used to control Crohn's disease symptoms. Luckily, science has come a long way since then, and there are many more choices currently available.

Corticosteroids are substances that resemble the hormones secreted by the adrenal glands. The adrenal glands are located on top of the kidneys, and the body produces corticosteroids by itself. This is true for all human beings, not just those with Crohn's disease. In fact, the human body probably produces the equivalent of about two and a half to three milligrams of prednisone a day. Corticosteroids like prednisone affect every cell in the body, and the body actually needs small amounts of them to sustain life. Prednisone is the most common and most well-known type of corticosteroid.

The advantages to taking prednisone include ease of administration and control of symptoms. It is administered orally and absorbed into the bloodstream. Prednisone can take anywhere from hours to days to take effect; it varies with each individual. For example, Jan a fifty-year-old woman who has had Crohn's disease for thirty-five years, has symptoms that wax and wane. When she is symptomatic (i.e., has diarrhea and abdominal cramping), she takes prednisone. She reports that she feels better within a few hours after taking it. However, Sam, a forty-two-year-old man who has had Crohn's for seven years, is also taking prednisone for his disease. He states that it takes at least a week for him to feel its effects.

Prednisone suppresses the inflammation in your intestine and all its manifestations (i.e., pain, fever, loss of appetite, weakness, fatigue, and abdominal tenderness). It is also used to suppress those difficulties that are found outside of the intestine, called *extra-intestinal manifestations*. Extra-intestinal manifestations include, but are not limited to, eye inflammation, skin rashes, arthritis, erythema nodosm (red, painful nodules on the legs), and pyoderma gangrenosum (an acute inflammatory bacterial dermatitis usually associated with ulcerative colitis). Prednisone helps these conditions, as well.

There are disadvantages to taking prednisone and many people do not like taking it as a result of those disadvantages. One disadvantage is that it suppresses normal adrenal gland functioning, which is why it can't be stopped abruptly. The adrenal glands need some time (days to weeks) to recover from the suppression induced by the prednisone and to return to normal functioning. Consequently, if your doctor wants you to discontinue prednisone, the daily dosage is tapered slowly, over time, rather than being abruptly discontinued.

Side Effects of Prednisone: Other disadvantages to prednisone include its many possible side effects. The side effects include fluid retention, or swelling of the face, hands, abdomen, and ankles. Some people's faces become especially swollen; the term for this is "moon face." If prednisone is prescribed for you, you might want to avoid foods high in sodium, as salt increases fluid retention. Also, fluid may collect around the back of your neck and cause your neck to appear swollen; this is referred to as a "buffalo hump." Prednisone can also cause sleeplessness, facial acne for both men and women, and for women, additional hair growth on the face is not uncommon. Other side effects include irritability, mood swings, crying spells, and for those taking prednisone for long periods of time or in high dosages, personality changes may result. Although these effects may sound horrible, they all disappear once the drug is stopped. It may help to remember that it wouldn't be prescribed if it didn't help.

Nevertheless, one of the major reasons people don't like to take prednisone is because of the side effects they tend to experience. It is noteworthy that different people react in varying ways to the drug. Some people don't get any side effects at all. Others get only a few side effects, and still others get almost all of them. You should also remember that once prednisone is stopped, all of the side effects disappear as well.

However, it is generally agreed that prednisone is not the drug of choice for long-term medical management of Crohn's disease. Physicians are aware of the drug's side effects, and they do not want you to be any more uncomfortable than you already are. If prednisone is the drug your physician prescribes, trust your doctor to know what's best for you, and be patient. Hopefully, you will feel better quickly and the side effects of the drug won't be an issue for you.

Methylprednisolone (Medrol) is the corticosteroid administered intravenously to people with Crohn's disease while they are in the hospital. It functions similarly to prednisone, except that it is administered directly into the bloodstream and is prescribed for those patients who, for example, may not be able to swallow medications while they are in the hospital.

On occasion, ACTH (adrenocorticotropic hormone) is used to stimulate the adrenal glands to produce their own steroids. In using ACTH to treat Crohn's disease, an effort is made to mimic and amplify the way the body's hormone system normally works. Today, as a rule, physicians do not employ this type of treatment. It was used when there were fewer medical options (i.e., drugs) available for physicians to prescribe.

There are also hydrocortisone-containing suppositories, enemas, and foamy aerols, which are available for topical rectal use. An *aerol* is foam that is used to treat disease of the rectum; it is also inserted into the rectum for treatment purposes. Suppositories are a method of transporting medication that is specifically prescribed because of the efficiency of transport. They are prescribed to treat disease in the rectal areas. Enemas are also prescribed for the efficiency of transport, but they are used to treat higher internal areas of the rectum. When inflammation is only in the rectum, or rectal area, medications such as these tend to be effective for reducing pain, inflammation, bleeding, and urgency.

Sulfasalazine (Azulfidine)

Sulfasalazine is used for mild to moderate Crohn's disease. It is a single drug that is comprised of a sulfapyridine component combined with a 5-aminosalicylic acid (5-ASA). It is administered orally. After an oral dose of sulfasalazine, approximately 25 percent of the drug is absorbed in the small intestine; the remainder passes to the colon where bacteria splits the chemical bond and releases the sulfapyridine and 5-ASA separately. The sulfapyridine acts as a "carrier," as it delivers the active portion of sulfasalazine, the 5-ASA component in its raw form, to the large, or lower, intestine. (The small intestine is sometimes referred to as the upper intestine; the large intestine is sometimes referred to as the lower intestine.) The sulfapyridine is absorbed and transported to the liver, where it undergoes a series of chemical reactions before it is expelled from the body in the urine.

Sulfasalazine is usually recommended for people who have Crohn's disease involving the colon. An average dose is approximately three to four grams/day (six to eight tablets). The side effects that people experience from sulfasalazine are most often due to the sulfapyridine component of the drug. Side effects are more likely to occur in higher dosages. These may include headaches, decreased appetite, and nausea, but usually reverse when the dosage is lowered (Peppercorn 1999).

Side effects are usually the result of a hypersensitivity or an allergic reaction and include rashes, fevers, nausea, vomiting, dizziness, lack of appetite, headaches, joint pain, and, rarely, hepatitis. For men, sulfasalazine may also cause a decrease in sperm count, which, like the other side effects, disappears when the drug is stopped. Sulfasalazine also impedes the absorption of folic acid, and supplemental folic acid may be suggested if you are taking it.

Sulfasalazine is an "older" drug. It was one of the first alternative medications to prednisone. It is unclear why sulfasalazine has beneficial effects in treating Crohn's disease. It does not prevent relapses of Crohn's disease that have been in remission, but when used as a maintenance medication, it can help you remain in remission. This medication is a sulfa-based drug (meaning that its composition has sulfa in it). There are some people who are allergic to sulfa, and cannot take this medication. Consequently, during the last ten to fifteen years, 5-ASA drugs were developed that are site-specific and do not contain the sulfa component. (Site-specific means that the drug is released in your digestive tract at a specific location.)

5-ASA Drugs (Aminosalicylates)

The drugs that were developed as alternatives to sulfasalazine, as a consequence of the sulfa component, are called the 5-ASA drugs. As previously stated, these drugs are site-specific and are released into different portions of the intestine. The type of 5-ASA prescribed for you depends on the location of your disease. Several forms of 5-ASA compounds have been developed.

Mesalamine (Asacol) is the 5-ASA compound that is released into the distal ileum and colon. Pentasa is released throughout the small intestine and colon. Olsalazine (Dipentum) and balsalazide (Colazide) are targeted for release in the colon. These drugs (5-ASAs) often must be used in larger dosages to achieve their maximum potential. Rowasa suppositories are 5-ASA topical medications that are used to treat the rectal area. Eliminating the sulfa component of sulfasalazine allowed 80 percent of those who could not tolerate sulfasalazine to take Mesalamine without experiencing ill effects (Peppercorn 1999). There are people, however, who do report some side effects. Rash, fever, and diarrhea are sometimes noted.

Immunomodulators

Immunomodulators affect the immune system by inhibiting the effects of T-helper cells (CD4 cells). CD4 cells are thought to play a role in the inflammatory aspect of Crohn's disease. Immunomodulators have been demonstrated to be effective in improving overall symptoms, including the healing of fistulas and allowing for the tapering off of steroids. They have also been effective in maintaining remission. 6-MP (Purinethol) and azathioprine (Imuran) are immunomodulators used for treating Crohn's disease.

These drugs, however, tend to be reserved for "steroid-dependent and drug-intolerant" people. Steroid dependent means that the body is dependent on steroids in order to maintain a minimum level of daily functioning. The person who is drug-intolerant has tried other drugs, such as 5-ASAs, and they have been ineffectual in treating the disease.

Cyclosporine

Cyclosporine, another type of immunomodulator, suppresses the immune system by blocking the effects of the CD4 cells on inflammation. It is used with transplant patients to assist in preventing organ rejection. Cyclosporine is effective for inducing remission in people who are not helped by other medications. However, there is a high relapse rate once the cyclosporine is stopped, and low dosages have not been found effective for maintaining remission (Peppercorn 1999).

Also, intravenous cyclosporine was demonstrated to be effective in inducing the closure of fistulas, but again, once the drug is withdrawn the fistulas recur. Cyclosporine should be avoided during pregnancy. Side effects of cyclosporine include increased growth of facial hair, numbness in the extremities (hands and feet), seizures, opportunistic infections, hypertension (high blood pressure), and kidney dysfunction. Blood levels should be monitored regularly while taking this medication.

Methotrexate

Methotrexate has been used for treating both rheumatoid arthritis and psoriasis, and has only recently been used with Crohn's patients. Its long-term effects are unknown as no controlled trials have been conducted to date. Methotrexate should not be taken during pregnancy. Because methotrexate is a relatively new treatment for Crohn's disease, potential side effects include but may not be limited to nausea, abnormalities in liver enzymes, and lowered white blood cell count.

Infliximab (Remicade)

Infliximab is a drug recently approved for use with Crohn's disease patients. It is given intravenously to those patients who do not respond to other medications. It is administered in a medical setting and does not require hospitalization. The reason infliximab is not commonly prescribed by physicians is due to the fact that it is very expensive. In addition, the long-term effects of the drug are unknown because of its "newness" on the market. To date, approximately 50,000 patients with inflammatory bowel disease and rheumatoid arthritis have received infliximab (Rogers 2000). Of those, an estimated 65 to 80 percent of patients with active Crohn's disease or another disease involving fistulas showed some improvement with an infusion of Remicade. Almost one-third of patients experienced a remission.

Interluken 10/11

Interluken 10/11 has not been approved for use with Crohn's disease patients in the United States. However, there are places in the country where the drug is being used for experimental purposes. There is not enough data at this point to state whether or not this drug is helpful in treating Crohn's disease. However, it is likely that it will be used in clinical experimental trials over the next several years.

Handling Emotional Reactions to Medications

It is not easy taking medications on a daily basis and it is not easy dealing with the side effects of those medications either. However, how you handle your reactions to taking medication can vary quite a lot, and a positive attitude about taking them can help you greatly. Regardless of the side effects you may or may not incur, you will have feelings about having to take medication routinely. It is important to remember that medications aren't your enemy, they are your helpers, or "medical friends," and if you let them, they can help you.

The mind is very powerful. You need to really believe that you are going to feel better, that your symptoms will pass, and that you will do whatever it is you want to do in life. The medications prescribed for you will help you achieve those goals. It is a natural reaction, however, to feel resentful, angry, sad, frustrated, and upset at the thought of having to take any medications at all.

Depression

At times, it is only natural to feel depressed when you have an illness that requires you to take medication regularly. It is a big adjustment to your lifestyle when you have to remember to take a bunch of pills every day, and taking them is far from pleasurable. For most people, swallowing pills wouldn't make the "Top 100 Things I Like to Do with My Day," even if it was ranked as number 100. So, when you are in one of those moods, you know, the mood that says, "So what if I miss my medication today? I just don't feel like taking it," or the mood that says, "This sucks. I just don't want to be reminded of it today," try to identify exactly what it is that bothers you about taking your medication, and what it is that makes you sad. Once you have identified what is making you sad and preventing you from taking your medication, ask yourself this: "What are the benefits and risks to my not taking my medication?" and "Who will I hurt in the long run?"

Although sometimes your sadness may result directly from the medication itself, it is more likely that the emotion stems from having to pop the pill in the first place. If that is the case, then you must try to fight the sadness, the frustration, and the anger. It is not your fault you have an illness that requires medication. When you become angry, frustrated, and/or sad and decide you need a break from your medication, you end up hurting only yourself. Instead of looking at the pills as reminders that you don't feel well, try to view them as "little helpers," who will assist you in achieving your goals, whatever they may be.

Taking medications can be even more upsetting when you are feeling well, and your doctor still wants you to take them. After all, you're feeling better, why take medication when you're not sick? It is at this juncture that you must be particularly aware of what you are feeling and thinking. For many people, this is a very vulnerable time. This is so because just as soon as you feel well, you want to forget that you have the disease, and move on with your life. For some people, forgetting they have the disease means forgetting to take the medications they are supposed to take to keep the disease in remission.

The fact is, if your doctor knows that you are feeling better, and he/she still wants you to take medications to maintain your remission, the chances are good that your doctor knows best. Some people may be able to forget about having the disease and can omit their medications for a while, even for many years (if they are lucky). But that doesn't change the fact that they have the disease. Whether you have symptoms or not, whether you take medications or not, you will always have the disease. Therein lies the sadness, the depression, the frustration, the anger, and the resentment you justifiably feel.

You do, however, have control over your emotions. You have control over your reactions and your thoughts and your behaviors. You can choose to be sad, frustrated, angry, and resentful—or you can choose an alternative. What alternative? The possibilities are limitless. You can feel, think, and behave in any way that you decide. You choose the feelings that you experience, as well as how to react to them.

Case Example: Adjusting Your Life

For instance, Sheila is a twenty-year-old woman with Crohn's who attends college and lives in the college dormitory. Her Crohn's disease is very active and, consequently, her physician prescribed multiple medications for her. She takes Asacol, Bentyl, prednisone, folic acid, and calcium supplements. Initially, she felt somewhat embarrassed at having to take so many pills, especially when her roommates saw her taking them.

But then she decided that she was not going to allow her illness to infringe on her interactions with others. She simply told her roommates, who had asked why she was taking so many pills, that she had Crohn's disease and the pills were her treatment. Sheila's roommates understood and were compassionate. To Sheila's pleasant surprise, they actually made jokes about her medical regimen, calling her "our druggie friend." Sheila made the use of her medications socially acceptable in the context of her social world. Consequently, adjusting her life to include medications became much easier.

Sleep Disturbances

Your disease activity can cause some type of sleep disturbance. So, knowing what to do about sleep disturbances is essential. There are drugs that may cause tiredness, and the chances are good that, if you are not feeling well, you are physically tired anyway. When you are tired, try to sleep as much as possible. Although it may be difficult to rearrange your schedule to get a few extra hours of sleep, it would be in your best interest to do so. Why? Sleep is healing; it gives the body time to rest and recuperate. Besides, the lack of sleep eventually will catch up with you, and at some time you will reap the consequence of sleep deprivation.

There are also drugs that can cause sleeplessness. You can be sleepless in the sense that you may have restless sleep, or you may not be able to sleep at all. Prednisone, for example, sometimes has that effect on some people. For instance, Arnold, a thirty-two-year-old man with Crohn's disease, was taking prednisone and couldn't sleep.

Long before Arnold started taking prednisone, his wife had stated that their house needed several repairs. Once he began taking prednisone and experienced difficulty sleeping, he painted their den and fixed anything and everything that was broken in the house, all between the hours of midnight and 6:00 A.M. Of course, ideally, you want to sleep in the middle of the night. He figured that if he was unable to sleep anyway, he might as well be productive. Once Arnold started feeling better, and the amount of prednisone was decreased, his sleep habits stabilized and became regular again. Arnold did not allow the ill effects of prednisone to hamper his attitude.

Readjusting Your Life to Include Medications

Medications help you by controlling the symptoms of your disease. They help quiet inflammation, promote healing of the diseased portions of your intestines, and improve the quality of your life. Most people respond well to carefully monitored and directed medical treatment and management. However, you have a right to participate in any decisions about your medical treatment. It is important for you and your doctor to identify those factors that worsen, or exacerbate, the disease activity in your body, and to eliminate those factors if at all possible.

It is within your rights as a patient to ask your physician why certain medications are prescribed, the details of their functions and benefits to you, the risks, side effects, and potential complications of the drug, as well as alternatives to its use. The more informed you are about your disease and the medications that you are taking, the more able you will be to understand your disease and yourself.

Taking Multiple Medications Simultaneously

If you are taking multiple medications for Crohn's disease simultaneously, your medical regimen should be monitored closely. If you are taking multiple medications for multiple medical problems, it is a good idea for your physicians to communicate with one another. Facilitating communication between multiple prescribing physicians ensures that you will receive the most appropriate and effective treatment, as well as assisting your physicians in understanding your medical difficulties. If you don't understand how multiple medications are helping you, ask the prescribing physician(s) to explain this to you, or to direct you to a source that will help in your quest for information.

What If You Stop Taking Your Medications?

As previously stated, you should think long and hard before stopping medications without the consent of your physician. However, there may be times when you do stop your medications. One such time might occur when you are on a maintenance dosage of a particular medication. If you are feeling better, why take drugs, right? Because *maintenance medication* is prescribed to help you stay in remission, or to keep you feeling well. It is very important that you tell your physician if you have stopped taking your medications. Why? This helps your doctor evaluate the disease activity in your body in an informed manner. If you don't tell your doctor that you have stopped taking your medication, your disease activity will be evaluated under the assumption that you *are* following the medical regimen prescribed by your doctor and he/she simply won't know what is really happening in your body.

Whether you are taking medications now or not, you need to be aware of the possibilities that exist and prepare yourself accordingly. The rest of part I discusses the possibilities of surgery, hospitalization, and the activities of daily living that may be affected by your disease. Just as this chapter may or may not apply to you, the following chapters should be read with equal caution, in the hope that your awareness of the various aspects of Crohn's disease will increase, regardless of your own personal experiences.

Chapter 4

Surgery:
The Reaper

"Baby take my hand. Don't fear the reaper. You can fly." These words are from the lyrics of a song entitled "The Reaper" by Blue Oyster Cult. Maybe you've heard this song before, maybe not. Although the words are not meant to refer to surgical cutting, in another context they might apply to you at some point in the course of your disease. If surgery is indicated for you, the recommendation will be made not to strike fear into your heart, but to help you feel better. Hopefully, you will never have to undergo an operation. But if you do, perhaps the words of this song will be a comfort to you.

Will you ever need an operation? Well, you may, and you may not. No one can predict with any certainty whether you will need an operation until the time you actually do need it. Approximately two-thirds of patients with Crohn's disease undergo surgery at some time during their lives (Sachar 1997). So it may be that you will fall into that 66 percent of the population. Surgery is one type of treatment for Crohn's disease. It is *not* a cure for it, even if all of the disease is removed from the diseased parts of your body.

If you do require surgery, the meaning of your operation and how you choose to deal with it is totally under *your control.* "Don't fear the reaper. You can fly." As previously stated, the only limitations you have are those you place on yourself.

This chapter discusses some of the surgical treatments for Crohn's, and also provides you with suggestions on *how to live* with Crohn's if you have to undergo an operation, or if you must be hospitalized.

Some people feel the worst part about Crohn's disease is that you never know what will happen next. Others choose to view such uncertainty as a part of the unpredictability of life. Everyone's perceptions vary and this influences the way in which all situations, not just operations, are viewed. The bottom line is this: surgery isn't pleasant for anyone at anytime, but how you choose to perceive the experience can help you deal with it, both in the moment and over the long term.

Overview of Surgical Treatments

Surgery is typically considered an appropriate treatment when medical treatments have been unsuccessful. In other words, if your Crohn's disease is active, and you have been taking medication that has not helped you, surgery is considered. You *don't* get told, "Hey, you have Crohn's disease, so go see the surgeon and have the disease in your body removed." That doesn't happen. So, if that is a fear of yours, don't worry about it. Surgery is recommended only when all other medical treatments have been tried and don't work. Moreover, surgery *is* invasive, both physically and emotionally, regardless of the cause, but you can choose to handle it in a manner that minimizes its invasive nature.

Surgery can be either elective or an emergency. In elective surgery, you choose to have the surgical procedure in order to improve your health and overall quality of life. In emergency surgery, there is no other option; you must have an operation to survive and function effectively. Having any type of operation for any reason can be frightening. After all, no one chooses to go into a hospital. Certainly, having your body cut open doesn't make your "Top Ten Things to do with My Day" list either. There are, however, ways to prepare yourself that will assist you before, during, and after surgical procedures.

Surgery for Crohn's Disease

There are several types of surgical treatments for Crohn's disease. The location of the disease in your body influences the type of operation that is most appropriate for you, which is another reason why you would want to know where the disease is located in your body. Again, remember that you may never need to have surgery; this is simply to inform you of the different surgical treatments available in the event that you or someone you know requires surgery for their disease. Also, some of the operations that are discussed certainly may occur for reasons other than Crohn's disease, such as ulcerative colitis or colon cancer.

Resection

A resection is a type of operation that removes the diseased portions of your intestine from your body. The remaining two ends of your intestines are then tied back together by the surgeon. The process of sewing the ends together is called *anastomosis*. Resection is one of the older surgical treatments (i.e., one that has been around for a while). A resection may be performed to remove a diseased portion of your intestine, or to treat internal fistulas.

An *internal fistula* is an abnormal opening in the intestine that leads to another part of the body. If an internal fistula has caused an *abscess* (infected area), the abscess is drained or removed. Incidentally, an abscess can also be external, and may feel as though you are sitting on a "black and blue mark," or a bruise (see chapter 3); it may look like a big zit around your rectal area. Resections are always done on an inpatient basis (that is, you must be hospitalized for this procedure), while draining external abscesses may be done on an outpatient basis. The final outcome of a resection is that after the surgery, the diseased portion of your intestine has been removed, and you can go to the bathroom in the same way that everyone else does. Resections are particularly appropriate for control of an abscess, in order to help the inflammation to heal.

When Cutting Helps

Daniel is a thirty-four-year-old man who has had Crohn's disease for ten years. Over the past several months, his disease has been quiescent, and he has not been on any medication. For about a two-week period Daniel thought he had bruised his rear end. He thought that he had hurt himself accidentally, and that was why he felt as though he was sitting on a "black and blue bruise." After approximately three weeks, Daniel inspected the area around his rectum. He wasn't feeling any better and he couldn't understand why the bruise hadn't disappeared yet. On inspection, he noticed a rather large, round, reddish swollen area, so he made an appointment with his physician. His doctor took one look and said, "You have an abscess, and I am going to drain it for you." The abscess was drained that same day, in the doctor's office. Fluid (which is why it was swollen and red) was drained from the area and Daniel was given a prescriptive ointment to sooth it. He felt much better afterwards.

The process of draining an abscess isn't pleasant. In Daniel's case, the physician, gave him a local anesthetic to numb the area, so that he could cut the skin and drain the pus from Daniel's behind. Doesn't sound like much fun, does it? However, as much as Daniel might not have wanted to have his abscess drained in that manner *in the moment*, the consequence was that after it was done, he felt much better almost immediately. Again, try to remember that physical pain in the moment may bring you physical relief over the long term.

Strictureplasty

A stricture is a narrowed portion of the intestine. In strictureplasty, the narrowed portion of the intestine is widened.

Strictureplasty is a slightly more complicated procedure than a resection. The ideal patient for strictureplasty is one with a short *stricture* and quiescent, that is to say, inactive, disease. In this procedure, an incision is made across the narrowed part of the intestine, and the intestine is surgically widened and sewn back together.

Because strictures are hidden due to the inherent curvature of the intestinal structure, it is sometimes difficult for physicians to discern how many strictures there are in the intestine. Typically, many strictures are found in the same general area of the bowel, and multiple strictures are fixed during the same operation. Contraindications for strictureplasty are perforation, abscess, phlegmon (suppurative inflammation and swelling), acute inflammation, and fairly long strictures (greater than fifteen centimeters). Strictures that are six centimeters or less are considered short strictures (Rolandelli 1994). When you've healed from a strictureplasty procedure, you defecate in the same way as all other human beings.

Ileoanal Anastomosis or Ileoanal Pouch Procedure

Ileoanal anastomosis is often referred to as a J-pouch or an S-pouch procedure. Although you might have heard of this procedure, it is not indicated for people who have Crohn's disease. Some people with ulcerative colitis require this procedure. This description is provided to increase your understanding of surgical procedures.

The type of name (J- or S-pouch) the surgery receives depends on the preference of the surgeon, as both operations are essentially similar. In the J-pouch procedure, the intestine is shaped similar to the letter "J"; in the S-pouch procedure, the intestine is shaped similar to the letter "S." That's the easy part of the explanation. An ileoanal anastomosis involves the following actions: The rectum and colon are removed and the anus and surrounding muscles are left in place. Then, the surgeon takes part of the small intestine and reshapes it (usually in a J or an S shape) to form an internal pouch, which functions as a rectum. After healing, it stores waste until you have to defecate. When people have this type of operation, they don't go to the bathroom any differently than they ever did.

In this procedure, however, a temporary ileostomy is sometimes created to allow the intestine to heal. A *temporary ileostomy* is a procedure that allows waste to pass into a pouch outside the body. The intestine heals during this time because waste is diverted to the stoma (an opening created outside the body from the intestine) where the waste is excreted into an external pouch, as opposed to traveling through the newly created J-pouch (rectum) inside the body.

Temporary ileostomies are not always performed with this procedure. It depends on the particular surgeon's approach to treatment. This type of operation is contraindicated for those with Crohn's disease, due to the chronic nature of the illness. In other words, because Crohn's disease frequently attacks other areas of the intestine, this type of surgery is contraindicated.

Proctocolectomy with Permanent Ileostomy

In this procedure, the colon, rectum, and anus are completely removed and the surgeon forms a stoma, from which waste can pass. A *stoma* is an opening located outside of the body that is created from the end of the small intestine (ileum), and sewn into the wall of the abdomen. It looks like an "outie" belly button with a hole in it. Because it originates from the inside of your body, it does not have nerve endings. When it heals completely, you can't necessarily feel when waste is excreted due to the absence of nerve endings. The outcome of this surgery is that waste passes from the small intestine to your stoma, where it is excreted and stored in a pouch, or bag, outside of your body, until you empty it.

Dealing with a permanent ileostomy. Living with a bag on the outside of your body is quite different from the outcomes of the other procedures described earlier because the manner in which you excrete waste is different. *It is not better or worse—just different.* The same rules still apply: The only limitations you have are those you place on yourself.

One of the most productive ways to help yourself adjust to living with an ostomy is to talk to other people who live with them. Although only a small percentage of people with Crohn's disease undergo ostomy surgery, many people who do not have Crohn's disease have ostomies for other reasons, such as colon cancer or ulcerative colitis. Contact the United Ostomy Association (UOA) as well as your local chapter of CCFA. Give them your number and tell them that you are interested in speaking to someone who has had experiences like yours. How to live with an ostomy is beyond the scope of this book; however, the same adjustment processes are involved as were discussed in chapter 1.

Continent Ileostomy

As a rule, a continent ileostomy, or Kock pouch, is performed on people who've had a permanent ileostomy, but who don't wish to wear an external pouch, or bag. This procedure is contraindicated for those with Crohn's disease, however, due to the risk of fistulas. Detailed information is provided here to increase your knowledge about surgical processes.

In this procedure, a segment of the small intestine is reshaped to form a pouch that holds waste inside the body. The internal pouch is connected to an opening in the abdominal wall, a stoma, to allow waste to leave the body. When you are healed from this procedure, waste collects within the pouch and it is drained from the stoma through a catheter (thin tube). A bandage covers the stoma when it is not in use to protect it. This procedure is most appropriate for those who have had a permanent ileostomy due to ulcerative colitis.

Anal Fistula Surgery

An *anal fistula* is an abnormal opening near the anus. Anal fistula surgery is a procedure wherein the fistula is surgically opened to help control infection, and to let nearby tissue and skin heal. Sometimes a stitch, or *suture*, is temporarily sewn in the fistula to allow an abscess to drain. This procedure can be done on an outpatient basis, whereas the other surgical procedures described above require hospitalization. If multiple fistulas with abscesses are present, multiple drains are placed to ensure that infections and complications do not arise.

Bypass Operations

Sometimes people with Crohn's disease may get abscesses on the inside of their bodies, usually in their small intestine. Bypass operations are used to drain an abscess that occurs on the inside of the body from one area of the intestine to another. Bypass operations require hospitalization.

Handling Hospitalizations

Spending time in the hospital is not on anybody's wish list. However, if you must, there are things you can do to make your life a little better. After all, if you have to spend time as a patient in a hospital, you might as well make the most of it. There are certain things you should know that will be of assistance to you, especially if you have never been hospitalized. The best way to handle hospitalizations is to prepare for them.

Preparing for the Hospital

Whether you are hospitalized for two days or two weeks, a certain amount of information will be of use to you during your hospital stay. First of all, you need to identify your expectations; what do you think it is going to be like? What do you expect will happen? How do you feel about it? In this manner, similar to the process discussed in chapter 1, you can alter your thoughts and feelings by changing your perceptions. You need to identify your feelings about hospitals, so that you can control any inclination to exacerbate negative emotions, such as fear or anger, which are emotions that will not serve you well during your stay in the hospital.

Identifying your expectations is helpful because if they are realistic, dealing with the hospital's physical environment, such as your room, your nurses, and the hospital's procedures will be easier to handle. For example, if you don't expect to get much sleep at all, you will be less affected by the nurses who come into your room in the middle of the night. If you have the expectation that your sleep will be undisturbed, you will make your time in the hospital more difficult than it has to be. Don't misunderstand, you *can* sleep well in a hospital (especially if you are given narcotics); it is just that if you *expect* to sleep soundly, your chances of being disappointed are that much greater.

Sleep, Privacy, and Respect

Don't expect to get a great deal of sleep, privacy, and/or respect while you are in the hospital and you will not be disappointed. Again, you most likely will get some sleep, privacy, and respect, at times. Nevertheless, certain hospital procedures can have a negative impact on you, if you allow them to be. Why is expecting to get well-rested sleep an unrealistic expectation? One reason was just mentioned, people will enter and exit your room all the time.

Many people share a room when they are hospitalized. Nurses come in and out of the room not just for your care, but also for the care of the person in the bed next to yours. The nurses will enter for various reasons, such as administering medication, checking blood pressure, and taking temperature. Furthermore, nurses change shifts three times in a twenty-four-hour period. Consequently, there will be several nurses whom you will see throughout the course of any given day. Your visitors and your roommate's visitors come and go as well. In addition, doctors enter and leave your room at random times throughout the day.

The physical logistics of the hospital affect your sleep, regardless of whether of not you are sharing a room. For instance, although most people sleep in the dark, the lights in the hallway are typically left turned on, and the doors to the hospital rooms are usually left open. Typically, a hospital has three shifts for its personnel: from 3 P.M. in the afternoon until 11 P.M. at night; from 11 P.M. at night until 7 A.M. in the morning; and from 7 A.M. in the morning until 3 P.M. in the afternoon.

Each shift of nurses, for example, typically will come into your room at least twice (when they come on duty and before they go off duty) to check your temperature and blood pressure. As previously mentioned, nurses also may come in and out throughout their shifts to administer medications, check your fluid intake, and/or fix your "attachments" (i.e., IV, heart monitors, etc.). Feel free to ask the nurses what medications you are taking as they are administered to you. Understanding what you are experiencing as it occurs will assist in decreasing and/or circumventing any anxiety you may feel.

Privacy and respect for patients can also be somewhat lacking in a hospital. Don't be upset if hospital personnel come in and out of your room without knocking. That is common hospital etiquette. Consequently, both privacy and respect can be lacking. However, if you expect to have very little privacy, you will be pleasantly surprised when you get some. There will be instances when you will have privacy, and there will be times when you feel respected. However, not expecting either privacy or respect prevents you from becoming frustrated when you don't have them. In this way, a stay in a hospital can provide you with a new and different appreciation for personal space, privacy, and respect for other human beings.

What to Bring

You will want to bring personal items that you need and that will make your stay in the hospital more comfortable. Although the hospital room will probably have a toothbrush, toothpaste, comb, etc., having your own personal things around you will make you feel better while you are there. Bringing basic personal items such as these, and perhaps cologne, or some other personal items that you like to have around you will bring a little feeling of "home" to an otherwise clean and sterile hospital room. You might also want to bring extra underwear or some of your own clothing to wear. If you do bring your own clothing, make sure that shirts, pajamas, sweaters, etc., are button-down types, as opposed to pullover items. Pullovers that go over your head won't work in a hospital if you need an intravenous (IV) drip.

Typically, people with Crohn's disease are placed on an IV drip that might be used for hydration, medication, and/or feeding purposes. If you are right-handed, you might consider placing the IV drip on the left or nondominant side of your body. Of course, if you are left-handed, you would reverse this. Such an arrangement will allow you greater freedom and flexibility when you are negotiating your movements around the room and bathroom. You may also receive a main IV line for feeding purposes in your shoulder or neck.

Bring materials that will occupy and/or amuse you that you can do by yourself, when no one else is around, or in the event that you can't sleep. You might bring books, crossword puzzles, cards, and/or crafts like knitting, crocheting, or sewing. A Walkman or Discman with some of your favorite music tapes and CDs will be helpful for many reasons. Music will help to divert your attention to something other than your illness and the hospital. Keeping your mind occupied with pleasant thoughts and diversions will be helpful to your entire healing process.

Hospital Personnel

Doctors and nurses are only some of the people whom you will encounter while in the hospital. Several physicians may visit you at one time. Your doctor may choose to bring teaching fellows and residents to look after you as well. This is the usual protocol at a hospital, especially teaching hospitals. When a group of white-coated people walk into your room, it does not mean that you are any healthier or sicker than you were two minutes before they arrived. It just means that your doctor (or someone else's doctor) is engaged in a round of teaching.

Doctors and nurses will not be the only people with whom you will interact during your hospitalization. Nutritionists, nurse's aides, and stomal nurses are other types of hospital personnel you may meet. Nutritionists who work for the hospital may be consulted to assist with planning your diet while you are an inpatient, as well as to help you plan an eating regimen to follow after your discharge. Nutritionists are particularly helpful while you are in the hospital because blood tests clearly demonstrate the specific nutrients your body needs. Nutritionists use this information to develop an eating plan specifically suited to your body's needs.

Stomal nurses are assigned to help people who undergo operations involving ostomies. They show you how the stoma equipment works, and how to use it in an effective manner for your lifestyle. They assist you with medical supplies and provide educational information to assist you in obtaining medical supplies from your health insurance carrier. (Note: Not all hospitals have stomal nurses.) Usually, the hospital initially provides you with medical supplies for surgery involving a stoma, as needed. The stomal nurse helps you to adjust during your postoperative period, which may occur on both an inpatient and outpatient basis.

While you are an inpatient in the hospital, you also might be visited by a psychologist or mental health clinician. Some physicians work in multidisciplinary settings, where various specialists treat you together to provide comprehensive treatment. Thus, a psychologist or mental health clinician might visit you, not because anyone thinks you are crazy, but to assist you emotionally, based on your needs at the time. For example, when Jennifer was in the hospital, she reported that she loved when the mental health clinician visited her. She said the psychologist listened to her vent all of her frustrations about being in the hospital. She also said that it made her feel better to have the chance to express herself.

Tips to Improve Your Hospital Stay

1. Don't expect to always get sleep, privacy, and/or respect. If you do get it, great, relish it.

2. Bring personal items like toothbrush, toothpaste, hairbrush, comb, cologne, soap, cosmetics, etc., to make your stay more comfortable.

3. Place the IV, if needed, on the nondominant side of your body.

4. Bring independent activities that you like to do to pass the time (i.e., music tapes or CDs, books, crosswords puzzles, etc.).

5. If you don't understand a process, ask questions.

6. Keep a journal and write down the information your doctor gives you so that you won't forget what you are told. Record any questions that you have, as well.

Preparing for Surgery

Just as there are specific actions you can take to prepare for hospitalization there are ways to prepare for surgery as well. Once surgery has been recommended to you, ask to speak to some people who have undergone the same procedures. You might want to ask two or three people. In this way, the individual differences and experiences among patients will be well illustrated, and you will be able to draw from multiple sources of information. Try to find out what were the most and least helpful experiences for these people, as this information may assist you as well.

The more information you have throughout the course of your illness, your hospitalization, and the surgical process, the better off you will be. Once you've gathered all your information, review it productively. That is, try to identify your feelings and thoughts about the procedure you are about to undergo. A major part of preparing for surgery is to prepare yourself emotionally.

Preparing for Hospitalization and Surgery

Victoria is a forty-four-year-old married woman who has had Crohn's disease since she was a teenager. Her physician has been recommending that she have surgery for several months. Initially, Victoria was completely against the idea. She had never had any type of operation, and she wasn't really interested in acquiring that kind of life experience. However, her physician suggested that she speak with some people who had received treatment similar to the surgery that was being recommended for her.

Victoria did that, and she was surprisingly encouraged by what she heard. Although no one she spoke to had enjoyed being in the hospital or having the operation, they all said that they felt better afterwards. Also, most of them added that their fearful anticipation had been worse than the actuality of the experience. The disease activity in her body wasn't improving, and so she decided to go ahead with the surgery.

Before arriving at the hospital, Victoria packed a bag to take with her to feel more comfortable. She took personal items such as toothbrush, hairbrush, cosmetics, shampoo, etc. She also took things that were meaningful to her, like a picture of her family and her journal. She wanted the journal so that she would be able to remember the questions that she had, and to record her feelings during the time surrounding her operation. Her husband and their children provided her with emotional and physical support during her hospitalization and postoperative period. Once the operation was over, Victoria was happy with her decision, and pleased that she had talked to the other patients because the information that she had received was indeed helpful.

Emotional Reactions to Your Operation

There are many emotions that you may experience both pre- and postoperatively. The entire surgical process (the hospital stay, the surgical residents and/or fellows, the preparation period, the anesthesia, etc.) are likely to influence some of your emotions. Conversely, your emotions are likely to influence how quickly you heal.

How Surgery Influences the Emotions

There is a wide range of feelings people normally have either in reaction to, or as a consequence of, the surgical process. The medications that you may be taking and the anesthesia that you are given just before surgery might also affect your emotional state. Although you may not think so, the combination of medications, anesthesia, and your own feelings can help or hinder your healing process.

Surgery Due to Medication Intolerance

Janet is a twenty-five-year-old woman who had to have an operation approximately six months after she was diagnosed with Crohn's disease. From the time of her initial diagnosis she experienced increased diarrhea and abdominal pain and was constantly losing weight. She didn't want to have surgery, but she wanted the diarrhea and the pain to stop. Medications were not effective, and her physicians thought that surgery was her best option.

Janet had never been hospitalized before and she didn't know what to expect either in the hospital or from the surgery. She was quite frightened and anxious; she was also quite ill physically. She cried frequently because she no longer had the emotional patience or tolerance for the physical pain. She didn't want to be in the hospital, but she didn't want to feel sick anymore either.

Janet was given anesthesia prior to her operation and noticed that she was attached to a morphine drip when she awoke. Postoperatively Janet said she still felt scared and out of sorts with herself, although she also felt relieved because she knew that she would be able to get better now.

Some of her emotional discontent was due to the anesthesia and the morphine. These substances made Janet feel quite hyper, that is, highly excitable and extremely fidgety, even with all the attachments she was hooked up to (i.e., catheter, IV drip, and morphine pump). Her physicians had to decrease the amount of morphine (which they would have done eventually, anyway). However, the decrease took place earlier than it otherwise would have because of the strong emotional reactions that Janet experienced.

Janet's reaction to the medications was such that her physicians recognized that the medications were altering her emotional status as well as her physical condition. Physicians pay attention to the quantity of medications you take—that's part of their job. In Janet's situation, the physicians tried to make her more comfortable by giving her the morphine, not realizing she would experience such an intense emotional reaction. Sometimes, both patients and physicians learn what is most helpful through trial and error. If Janet ever requires surgery again, she and her physicians will choose a different pain medication postoperatively.

How the Emotions Influence Surgery

Just as the surgical process can influence your emotions, your emotions can have an impact on your healing process. The way your feelings affect your adjustment to your disease is similar to the way they impinge on your adjustment to an operation. If you are very anxious and fearful prior to your surgery, your experience will be quite different than if you are emotionally ready and relaxed (that is, as relaxed as you can be) prior to your surgery.

The range of possible emotions was discussed in chapter 1. Denial, fear, anger, anxiety, and sadness are all normal feelings when you are first diagnosed with any chronic illness. This is also true when you have to undergo an operation—any operation, regardless of whether it is a consequence of Crohn's disease or not.

Do operations for Crohn's disease influence your emotions any differently than operations for other reasons? Probably not. Fear and anger, anxiety and depression are all natural responses that you may feel in situations that involve invasive procedures. The steps listed in chapter 1 can be helpful to you when undergoing surgery, as well as when dealing with chronic illness.

Identify your thoughts and your feelings. Become aware of what it is that is most upsetting and distressful to you, so that *you can help yourself.* Don't let feelings of fear, anxiety, depression, and anger debilitate you. Identify your feelings, acknowledge them, and then take action to alter those that aren't working for you, or are hindering you. Although this is much easier to say or to write than to put into practice, you've been able to read this book this far. You are learning ways to help yourself in an undesirable situation right now, as you read this. Whether you are currently feeling physically and/or emotionally well or not, reading this book is proactive. You've taken the initiative and have had the courage to read about some unpleasant things. Hopefully, you will never have to use the material in this chapter. But if you do, try to remember that you will be okay and that you are not alone.

Activating your support system when you need to have an operation is always a good idea. Chapter 9 is devoted to social support. Reaching out to the people you love, who love and care about you, is always helpful in stressful situations, especially when you don't feel physically well. Prepare the people you want to be around you. Tell them only what you feel comfortable with sharing. Let them know when you will be in the hospital and what you will need from them. See chapter 7 for a discussion on how, who, why, and when to share your illness.

Surgery for Alan

Alan is a fifty-seven-year-old married man who was diagnosed with Crohn's disease when he was in his mid-thirties. Initially, his disease was well controlled with medication. Alan's disease went into a remission that lasted for about twelve years. During that time he did not take any medication nor did he experience the gastrointestinal symptoms of Crohn's disease. However, in the past several years,

Alan's disease had become active again. He was taking medication and had developed an obstruction, or blockage, in his intestine that required surgery.

Due to the acute nature of the situation, Alan could not prepare as much as he would've liked. He had all he could do to adjust to the idea that he was going to have an operation. He called his family, his children, and those people at his office whom he needed to notify. He also called a few of his close friends who knew that he had Crohn's disease and told them what was happening, because he knew that they would be emotionally supportive. Having his family and friends around after surgery was helpful to him because it took his mind off of his body for a while and provided him with other people and situations to consider. Also, the many visitors he had helped him to pass the time in the hospital prior to his discharge.

Tips for Surgery

1. Speak to at least one individual who has had the operation that you will have.

2. Ask what the person's experience was like (i.e., What was most helpful? What was least helpful?).

3. Make sure your health insurance carrier has the appropriate authorizations and necessary referrals.

4. If time allows, prepare everything that you will need in the hospital in advance.

5. Call the people who need to be notified (employers, family, etc.) and prepare and activate your support system.

6. Designate a guardian ad litem.

7. After surgery, hold a pillow over your incision when you rise, sit down, cough, and/or sneeze to minimize physical pain.

8. Use an inner tube (from a bicycle tire) to sit on, if necessary, to minimize pressure on your buns (if that's where the surgery was performed).

Alternative Treatments

Alternative treatments are all those treatments not based on western allopathic medicine and science. Meditation, reiki, fish oils, etc., are all forms of alternative treatments. The various types of alternative treatments available are beyond the scope of this book. Moreover, alternative treatment used as "alternatives" to standard medical treatments for people with Crohn's disease can be dangerous to your physical health. Using such alternatives as supplemental to medical treatments *with your physician's knowledge* is okay.

Today, alternative treatments are the subject of much controversy among the medical profession. Discuss those treatments in which you are interested with your doctor. It will improve your relationship with your doctor, as well as informing you of what appropriate options exist. Discussing these matters with your physician will also ensure that you won't do anything to hurt yourself.

For example, a twenty-nine-year-old man, George, had active Crohn's disease and was looking for any way to feel better. He was taking medication but he didn't feel that it was helping his physical symptoms of diarrhea and abdominal pain. He heard about someone with a Ph.D. in nutrition, who was providing "alternative treatment" to people with medical illnesses. George called and made an appointment to see him. At his appointment, which consisted only of a physical examination, he was told to take several types of vitamins and minerals, and to drink a liquid form of aloe three times a day. George followed this regimen. After a few days, he had to call his regular physician because his physical symptoms had worsened considerably.

When he kept his appointment, George told his doctor about his visit to the person with the Ph.D. in nutrition, and of the substances that he was ingesting. George's doctor told him that the aloe might be causing the increase in his diarrhea and cramping. The doctor told him to stop taking the aloe immediately. When he did, his pain subsided and the number of times he had to defecate decreased. Was it definitely the aloe that caused his symptoms to increase? There is no certainty of that. But in George's case, the aloe clearly didn't help him either.

Whenever you ingest something that differs from your daily routine and habits, pay attention to the manner in which it affects you (if at all). Chapter 10 deals directly with nutrition and eating patterns.

Now that both medical and surgical treatments of Crohn's disease have been considered, the following chapters will deal with how to live with the physical symptoms of Crohn's.

Chapter 5

Coping with Physical Symptoms

Now you have some background on how Crohn's disease may affect you physically, including information on both the medical and surgical treatments available to you. Hopefully, you also have a greater understanding of some of your thoughts about your illness and your feelings surrounding it, as well as understanding why the relationships you establish and maintain with medical professionals are important to your physical and emotional health.

The first part of this chapter focuses on what you can do to make your day-to-day life more tolerable when your disease is active, as well as what you can do to circumvent difficult situations that may arise during the activities of day-to-day life. The second half of the chapter provides you with a variety of ways to deal with chronic pain, including different coping strategies and relaxation methods. Although these strategies may apply to you as someone living with Crohn's disease, you also may find them useful for situations unrelated to your disease.

Daily Life

Living with Crohn's disease may become difficult, especially when the disease is active. For those with inactive disease, life on a daily basis is probably not that different from anyone else's. For example, your diet may be slightly different from that of your family, peers, and coworkers, or it may not. Changing your eating habits affects only you, and is usually unnoticeable, unless you live with another person.

If your disease is inactive, you can live without having to share your diagnosis with anyone. No one will be likely to notice your slightly different eating habits or the frequency with which you use the toilet. Moreover, if your disease isn't active, it is not affecting your daily routine and habits. For those of you with active disease, however, daily life can be an entirely different matter.

There are several reasons why living with Crohn's disease is challenging when your disease is active. One is that although everyone, every human being you know, defecates, it is a topic rarely discussed in conversation. Consequently, explaining that life is difficult for you because you have to use the bathroom more than most people doesn't make much sense to most of the "healthy" people in your life. Sometimes, people have difficulty understanding why having frequent diarrhea is debilitating, because most people have had diarrhea, too, at some point in their lives.

Hence, living with Crohn's disease may be troublesome because the symptoms of the disease are taboo for discussion. You may find it both stressful and arduous to discuss society's unspeakable topic. (A detailed discussion of how and when to disclose such information is provided in chapter 7.) Having a socially unacceptable illness where secrecy is commonplace can make living with it much more burdensome for you than it needs to be.

There are, however, ways to make living with Crohn's disease easier for yourself. You may choose to share with others, or not, that is your choice. After all, you have to live with the disease, why should you have to talk about it too, right? It is, however, always more helpful to communicate with your loved ones about what is happening in your life, regardless of whether or not it involves defecation. Nevertheless, you need not share the information if you don't wish to. Be advised that withholding such information can make life a bit more complicated for you than it needs to be. For now, the information provided is to assist you in the activities of day-to-day living.

Social and Occupational Activities

Pursuits such as work, school, relationships, parties, exercise, and such, those events and situations which comprise your daily life, can be influenced by your disease process. For example, in any given day, you wake up and begin your daily routine. Perhaps you prepare and take your children to school, perhaps you go directly to work, and perhaps you do both. Regardless of your daily activities, active Crohn's disease can, and frequently does, alter your routine.

For example, James is a twenty-six-year-old accountant who must be at work by 8:30 A.M. daily. His Crohn's disease tends to be more active in the mornings (i.e., he has diarrhea mostly in the mornings). When he was first diagnosed with Crohn's, James used to arrive almost a half hour late to work each day because of his morning bowel habits; he simply could not get off the toilet to make it into the office on time. James' boss was becoming irritated with him for his continual tardiness, so, consequently, James started getting up earlier in the morning. He arose a half hour earlier each day to accommodate both his bowels and his boss. He changed his daily routine to accommodate his lifestyle in the context of his disease. He also chose not to share the information about his illness with his boss.

This illustrates how you can go through your daily activities and not tell people what is going on with you. James could have chosen to tell his boss about his illness, and his boss might have had a different response to his tardiness. Perhaps his work schedule would have been changed to accommodate his disease, instead of the other way around. Or perhaps his boss would not have been irate at all. You can't predict how others will react to hearing about Crohn's. See chapter 8 for a discussion of some of the reactions that others may have to your disease.

Throughout each day certain situations will arise that you can expect, as will situations that are totally unexpected. Preparing in advance will help you to feel more comfortable in all kinds of situations. For instance, you might have noticed your increased awareness of where bathrooms are located throughout the places you frequent in your daily life; this appears to be a common trait among people who have Crohn's disease. Why? Knowing where the bathroom is located helps to decrease anxiety and makes you feel more secure, just in case the need arises.

Using humor is another way to decrease anxiety and alleviate tension; it also makes a socially unacceptable topic more acceptable.

Jill, for instance, is a twenty-one-year-old woman with Crohn's disease who frequents nightclubs on weekends with her friends. Her stomach usually doesn't cooperate with her social plans, as she frequently needs to defecate. Hence, she jokes with her friends about her frequent need for a bathroom.

Jill says, "You know the movie *Where the Boys Are*? Well, my stomach wants to know, 'Where the Bathrooms Are!'" Through the use of humor, Jill is able to communicate her needs in a way that is readily accepted by her peers. Her friends simply don't care if she needs a bathroom more often than they do, they care about her and want her to take care of her physical needs.

Expected Situations

There are certain situations you can prepare for in advance. Expected situations are those situations where you know that your disease process may have an influence on your behavior. Traveling, parties, and/or work-related situations, such as taking clients out to lunch or dinner, are examples of situations where bathroom location and eating and drinking habits may influence your behavior and/or coping with your disease. Preparing for such situations or having a plan of action is helpful for both your physical and emotional sense of well-being.

Traveling by Car

Whether by car, train, airplane, or boat, traveling can be burdensome for you if you have active Crohn's disease. Driving either short or long distances can produce anxiety, especially when you are in unfamiliar areas. For instance, Michael, a forty-two-year-old man sells radio airtime to earn his living. His job requires him to spend much of his day in his car, and to wine and dine potential buyers. He can tell you the cleanest bathrooms along Interstate 95 for the sixty-mile area that he travels regularly.

When you spend much of your time in a car, whether it is due to occupational reasons or not, it is always good to identify potential places to stop and use the rest room along the way. Fast food restaurants generally have clean rest rooms, and they are easily located off major roadways. If you know you will be driving long distances, you may wish to carry an extra pair (or two) of underwear with you in your trunk. Michael has had many bouts of active Crohn's disease throughout his lifetime. Due to his heavy traveling schedule, as well as the fact that his disease, when active, tends to be severe, he used to carry a portable "potty" in his trunk, just in case he wasn't near a place he could stop and use a toilet. It alleviated the stress of not knowing whether a bathroom would be available for him to use or not.

Traveling by Airplane

Traveling via airplane can also cause anxiety. In addition to the physical confinement, the bathrooms are limited in number. Again, preparing in advance for the flight can help decrease your anxiety and stress level. For instance, if you know that your bowels are active in the morning, you can schedule afternoon or evening flights. In other words, try to schedule flights at a time when your bowel is least active.

Since this may not always be possible, and/or your bowel may not cooperate with your flight travel, go to the bathroom just before you board the airplane, regardless of whether you really need to use it. Also, if you know that your bowels are more active when you have eaten, don't eat prior to the flight time. Temporarily adjust your eating habits to accommodate your bowel habits in the context of flying. If the flight is going to be unusually long, and you know that at some point you *will* have to use the rest room, carry your own toilet paper or tissues, which may be softer than the type of paper the airplane provides.

Traveling Abroad

Traveling abroad can be a wonderful experience and, hopefully, need not be hindered by your disease. Depending on where you are traveling, bathrooms tend to be equally as clean, if not more so. If you are nervous about the quality of the toilet paper, bring your own. Also, the water abroad can influence your bowels, not because you have Crohn's disease, but because water abroad can influence anyone's bowel habits. It is easy to pick up Montezuma's revenge, or diarrhea, when you are traveling. Try to drink only bottled water, either buy your own or bring some with you. Bottled water is sold wherever you travel. Be responsible and cautious. If you know that certain foods eaten at home increase your diarrhea, don't eat them while you're away.

Another way to prepare for traveling abroad is to consult with your physician. If your disease is active during the time you plan to travel, prior to leaving consider asking your physician if he knows of a physician or hospital you can go to (if it becomes necessary) in the geographic area to which you are traveling. In the event of an emergency, you will have a predetermined place or person to contact, recommended by your physician.

Traveling by Boat

Boat rides can present unique challenges for all people, not just those with Crohn's disease. There's always the chance that the water may be rough and seasickness can arise, which can upset anyone's stomach. Consequently, cruises on large ships may not be your idea of an ideal vacation. Traveling on smaller private boats may be something that you'd like to do, but fear, due to the uncertainty of your stomach. Not all private boats have toilets, do they? And when they do, they're often small, and the person whose boat you're traveling on has to clean it.

You should never do something that you're not comfortable with as it will increase your anxiety and stress level. The fact is you always have choices. You can choose to accommodate your eating and drinking habits such that you won't need to use the bathroom during a boat ride (or on an airplane ride for that matter). You simply can avoid going out on boats all together, which would be a shame, since many people find it to be a really enjoyable, fun activity.

In a situation such as this, for example, disclosure of your illness would probably be helpful to you. If you tell the person whose boat it is that you've got Crohn's disease, it may make it easier for you. Why? Because then you simply ask that person to stop somewhere so you can use a real toilet, instead of the one on the boat. It is fairly likely that the boat owner will accommodate you. But if you're really uncomfortable with the idea of being on the water, just don't do it. As with any other activity, if you are uncomfortable in a situation, you won't enjoy yourself.

Parties

Why might private parties require preparation? Well, they are usually held in someone's house, with a limited supply of toilets. If there are a limited number of bathrooms available, and many people are waiting to use the rest room, odors and smells can be embarrassing, especially for you. After all, who wants to use a rest room where there's a line, and the next person to use the toilet actually will know you've used it? In these situations, you might use the rest room least likely to be visited by guests (like the one in the master bedroom). Again, you might want to cut down or alter your eating and drinking habits to decrease your need to use it. For example, if drinking alcohol exacerbates your diarrhea, don't drink it. With larger parties held at hotels, restaurants, catering halls, etc., you may not encounter such difficulties, as rest rooms are typically available and plentiful. You might also carry a book of matches around with you. When you've finished using the rest room, strike a match; the sulfur assists in eliminating odors.

Unexpected Situations

Because you have a disease that involves the digestive system, relief from abdominal pain and cramping may manifest itself in ways other than defecation. For instance, burping and passing gas can relieve abdominal pain and cramping, as well. Two activities, unfortunately, that may not be uncommon to those of you with Crohn's. Of course, when people discuss such activities, it is usually in the form of a joke, and usually in a derogatory context. You may have a greater appreciation of such jokes, though. Perhaps you don't think they are so humorous either. Maybe you don't have difficulty burping and/or passing gas in public places. Perhaps it doesn't bother you at all.

However, most people, regardless of whether they have Crohn's disease or not, become self-conscious when they pass gas or burp. Why? Well, generally speaking, bodily odors and smells aren't attractive. For women, such odors certainly aren't considered feminine and such activities are more embarrassing than they are for men because of the social stigma inherent in burping and passing gas. For men, such activities aren't any less embarrassing or likable, but they are just slightly more acceptable by society.

Burping

Linda is a twenty-seven-year-old woman who has had Crohn's disease since her freshman year of college. Most of her close friends are aware that she has Crohn's disease, and she has been sick on and off since her diagnosis. Currently, her disease is quite active and she has difficulty digesting almost all kinds of foods. Her stomach is frequently empty, and as a consequence, she burps a great deal.

Linda has told her friends that she gets easily embarrassed when she feels the need to burp, especially because she does it with such frequency. After Linda's disclosure to her friends, they began to make jokes about the entire process in a positive manner, which helps Linda feel more comfortable. Linda says that when she and her friends go out to eat, they tease her. They say things like, "Okay, everybody, who can guess how many times Linda will burp after she finishes eating?" Linda reports that her friends have made her feel much better about her behavior. This illustrates how both self-disclosure and using humor in uncomfortable situations places an otherwise unacceptable social behavior into a different context.

Handling Gas

Passing gas is a bodily function that everyone engages in at one time or another. You don't have to have Crohn's disease to pass gas. If you do have Crohn's, you simply may be more likely to do so. How can you deal with it? The same way everyone else does. You excuse yourself and leave the room (if you can). If not, well, you just have to live through it, as will the people in the surrounding areas. Just as everyone you know defecates, all human beings also pass gas.

There are ways to decrease the frequency with which you pass gas. For instance, some foods make passing gas more likely to occur than others. Onions, mushrooms, raw vegetables, and spicy sauces are foods likely to increase such behaviors among most people, which means that avoiding these foods may apply especially to you. Also, if you find that passing gas is particularly troublesome, discuss it with your doctor. Your doctor should know if you're passing gas frequently, anyway.

Having Accidents

If you have ever been afraid of having an accident, you are not alone. Most people with Crohn's disease have that fear at one time or another. If you have active disease, it may be that you might not be able to control your bowels. You may indeed "have an accident," which, incidentally, would not be the end of the world. One way to decrease the anxiety engendered by this particular fear is to carry extra underwear around with you. Keep it in your car, bag, at a desk drawer at work, wherever you will have easy access in case you need to use it. In the worst-case scenario, you throw your soiled underpants away, and put on the clean ones. Remember that "having an accident," while certainly unpleasant, may be a consequence of active disease. It does not mean that you've behaved badly (as you were taught when you were two years old).

What to Do About Chronic Pain

If you have active Crohn's disease, chronic pain is a problem that may arise for you. The pain may increase or decrease depending on the disease activity in your body, the amount and type of food you eat, and how frequently you use the bathroom. Try to remember that your disease process, like you, is unique. Some people experience pain prior to and during defecation only. Other people experience pain with the active disease regardless of whether they have eaten anything or not. Some of you may experience pain only when you eat. Others may not experience any physical pain at all.

In an ideal world, the way to eliminate your physical pain permanently would be to eliminate the disease. In the real world, this is not possible. When you are in pain all the time, it can be very debilitating. You may feel frustrated, angry, intolerant, and impatient simply because you are in physical pain. Consequently, learning ways to manage your pain can be very helpful to you. The next section of this chapter provides you with ways to decrease or alleviate the physical pain you may be experiencing.

There are many different ways to manage chronic physical pain. Some of you may choose to treat pain with medication, some of you may not. Several ways to treat chronic pain will be discussed here. Medications will not be discussed in detail (see chapter 3 for more details on medications).

Visualization and/or guided imagery, for example, are two relaxation methods that are also used for chronic pain management; they may or may not work for you. Only you know what helps to alleviate your physical pain fast. To figure out which pain management technique is most helpful to you, you need to try them out. Not all techniques will be helpful to you; some will work better for you than others, some you will enjoy more than others, and that's okay. The idea is to figure out how to manage your physical symptoms in such a way that it promotes your physical and emotional well-being.

Medications

Medications may be used to manage pain, with your physician's knowledge. Sometimes, medications like Bentyl, a muscle relaxer, or Percocet, an opiate, may be prescribed for your pain. However, due to the chronicity of your physical symptoms and to the risk you take in becoming drug-dependent, you may want to try using other forms of pain management, such as pain diaries or relaxation methods, which are described below. Medications may alleviate your physical pain in the moment, but the long-term effects of taking medication for pain management purposes may not be in your best interests.

Pain Management Techniques

Physical pain manifests itself in both your physical behavior and your thoughts. Pain may influence your behaviors, like remaining in bed when you're in pain, staying home from work and/or school, making facial expressions, guarding your movements, or complaining verbally (Keefe and Beckham 1994). Beliefs, expectations, attitude, and attentional focus also can influence your perception of and reactions to your physical pain (Chapman 1978; McCaul and Malott 1984).

Pain Diaries

Keeping a pain diary, a recording of pain and related behaviors and thoughts, is one way to increase awareness of your physical pain and relieve it by changing your behaviors and thought patterns. In a pain diary, you keep a record of when you have pain, the medications you take for it, your activity level, and your perception of the environment at the time (Keefe and Beckham 1994).

When you keep a pain diary, you rate the amount of pain you experience on a scale (typically on a scale of one to ten, with ten meaning unbearable, and one as barely noticeable). In addition, you should record the activity you are engaged in at the time of experiencing the pain. Ideally, you want to keep a pain dairy so that after you form a sense of when you have pain, and what you think about it, you can alter your perceptions of the pain, and your behaviors surrounding it.

You want to be able to recognize the relationship among your thoughts, your behaviors, and your feelings of pain. For example, you may read this and say to yourself, "I will never be able to cope with all the pain I feel." This statement is an example of *catastrophizing*, or an exaggerated statement of the truth. It may be very difficult for you to cope with physical pain, but you are dealing with it (even though you may not think so). Positive self-affirmations and self-reflection are ways to manage such cognitive distortions.

Self-affirmations

Positive self-affirmations are statements that will help you deal with your pain, both physically and emotionally. They can help you with things you want to do, such as cope with your pain, or deal with a problem you are facing. For instance, in the example above, you might change the statement to "I am really hurting, but I can deal with it." If you wanted to control your pain, you might say, "I can handle the pain; it is not that bad." In this context, positive self-affirmations also can be used for purposes other than pain management.

For example, if you wanted to achieve better control over your temper, you might say to yourself, "I have control over my temper" or "I will control my temper so that I can have a better relationship with my partner." The positive affirmations that you choose for yourself should be short, convincing, realistic, and something that you can control. For example, "I'm going to be on the television show with Regis and win a million dollars" would not be a good choice because it is not realistic. However, saying to yourself, "I will take my medication every day" is a behavior that you can control.

Relaxation Techniques

Relaxation training is probably one of the most frequently employed treatments for pain. There are several different kinds of relaxation exercises (Keefe and Beckham 1994). This section of this chapter will introduce you to a few of the most common forms of relaxation techniques. Most people, regardless of whether they have Crohn's or not, have a preference. Which method is best for people who have Crohn's disease? The method that works best for you, regardless of the kind of technique it is. How will you know what is best? Try a few different types and see which works well for you and which you find most enjoyable. A relaxation technique works well when it accomplishes its goal: helping you to feel relaxed and at peace with yourself. The idea is to establish and maintain an inner peace within yourself. Relaxation techniques can assist you in achieving that goal.

You do not have to use the relaxation techniques described in this chapter. They are provided to you as examples of what some people find helpful. There are many who choose to practice relaxing in nontraditional ways, such as in a hot bath listening to music, or taking yoga classes, or meditating. Daily relaxation, for however long you choose to relax, is helpful to your own sense of inner peace, which makes it easier for you to handle anything that comes your way—including the activity of your disease.

Diaphragmatic Breathing

Diaphragmatic breathing is one very popular way to help you relax. Breathing is one of the easiest ways to release tension and induce relaxation. It is the physiological system you can control most easily (Antoni and Schneiderman 1998; Antoni, Schneiderman, and Ironson 2000). When you feel stress, anxiety, or tension, you are usually breathing through your upper chest. For some of you, breathing through your upper chest may have become so habitual that it replaces your natural, diaphragmatic breathing. Shallow breathing actually perpetuates tension (Antoni and Schneiderman 1998; Antoni, Schneiderman, and Ironson 2000). If you have ever watched how a sleeping puppy breathes, you will have noticed that the puppy's abdomen moves up and down with each breath. This is an example of diaphragmatic breathing.

Exercise: Diaphragmatic Breathing

First find a comfortable position for yourself. Diaphragmatic breathing can be practiced anywhere, as long as you are comfortable. Notice how you are breathing when you first begin to practice. Hold one hand over your chest and one hand over your stomach, and then just breathe naturally. If the hand over your chest is moving up and down, you are not breathing from your diaphragm, you are breathing through your chest. You know that you are breathing through your diaphragm when the hand on your stomach is moving up and down. As you begin to inhale, take a deep breath from your abdomen, hold it for a few seconds and then exhale. As you exhale, you should see your abdomen move outwards. When you are used to shallow breathing (as most of us are), diaphragmatic breathing takes some practice. Counting to the count of 3 as you inhale, holding to the count of 3, and exhaling to the count of 3 will help you to monitor your speed, and slow you down if you are breathing too quickly.

When practicing diaphragmatic breathing, posture is important because it facilitates the motion that your diaphragm makes when you are breathing this way. In addition, counting to yourself as you breathe in and out will help you to monitor your pace. Diaphragmatic breathing can be practiced anywhere: in a car, watching television, or waiting for your children to come out of school. The key to successful relaxation, including diaphragmatic breathing, is to practice it.

Autogenic Training

Autogenic training (AT) is another way to relax. It is a method of relaxing that involves repeating different phrases to yourself. You can use autogenic training for any part of your body, including slowing down your breathing and slowing down your heartbeat. The idea behind autogenic training is to become peaceful, calm, relaxed, and serene with yourself. In autogenic training, you repeat relaxing self-suggestions to different parts of your body. You may begin with any body part you wish: arms, legs, forehead, etc. Some people prefer to start with their extremities such as arms and legs. Others start with the top of their heads and progress downwards (forehead, head, neck, etc.). The idea is to practice the exercise in a manner that makes you feel most comfortable, regardless of the order of the body parts you choose to relax.

Exercise: Autogenic Training

When you practice autogenic training, like diaphragmatic breathing, you should do it in a comfortable position in a quiet and relaxing environment. Each phrase should be repeated; ideally, from four to five times. You may choose to start with any part of your body that you wish, as long as you know that you are developing a pattern that works for you. That is, you don't want to practice autogenic training differently each time you do it. You might start with the body parts that collect the most tension. For some people, this may be their head and neck, for others their arms and legs. The following statements are some self-suggestions that are used in autogenic training. Each statement should be repeated to yourself several times.

My forehead is cool.

My neck and face are warm.

My neck and face are heavy.

My neck and face are warm and heavy.

My shoulders are warm.

My shoulders are heavy.

My shoulders are warm and heavy.

My right forearm is warm.

My right forearm is heavy.

My right hand is warm

My right hand is heavy.

My right hand and forearm are warm and heavy.

My left forearm is warm.

My left hand is warm.

My left forearm is heavy.

My left hand is heavy.

My left forearm and hand are warm and heavy.

I feel calm and relaxed.

My breathing is calm and regular.

My torso is relaxed.

My left thigh and leg are warm.

My left thigh and leg are heavy.

My left foot is warm.

My left foot is heavy.

My left thigh, leg, and foot are warm and heavy.

My right thigh and leg are warm.

My right thigh and leg are heavy.

My right foot is warm.

My right foot is heavy.

My right thigh, leg, and foot are warm and heavy.

I am peaceful and serene.

When you are ready to stop this exercise, repeat to yourself: *"I am alert and refreshed."* Remember to continue to practice your breathing throughout this exercise.

With practice, you will become increasingly better at this exercise. Practicing will help you to become more deeply and completely relaxed. Every time you practice, your desire to control your tension will increase, and you will be able to relax more quickly (Antoni and Schneiderman 1998; Antoni, Schneiderman, and Ironson 2000). The effects of the calmness and relaxation you attain may carry over to the other parts of your life throughout your day. You will feel calm and relaxed, and be aware of tension or excess energy whenever it manifests itself.

Progressive Muscle Relaxation

Progressive muscle relaxation (PMR) is a form of relaxation that makes you more aware of the tension in your muscles. In PMR, you learn how to tense and relax your muscles in order to decrease or ease the amount of tension in your different body parts. When your muscles are relaxed, it relieves tension in your body. For instance, when you make a fist, you feel tension in your muscles. When you release the fist, you feel your muscles relaxing.

In PMR, you pay attention to both the feelings of tension and relaxation as they occur. By practicing this exercise, you will increase your awareness of the tension in your body across all situations, not just when you are practicing. By becoming aware of the tension in your body, you can learn to reduce it using the relaxation methods described here.

Exercise: Progressive Muscle Relaxation

Again, you want to practice this exercise by lying down or sitting in a comfortable position. Practice your breathing first. Once you've spent a few moments breathing through your diaphragm, begin the exercise.

Because the idea of PMR is to notice the difference between tension and relaxation, you will need to tense the muscles in your body, hold the muscles in a tense position, and then release the muscles and relax them.

First, concentrate on your facial muscles, your eyes, nose, mouth, and chin. Tense all these facial muscles and hold it (make a funny clown face, crinkle your nose, squint with your eyes, etc.). Hold the tension for about three to five seconds and release it. Notice the difference between the tension and the relaxation. Tense the muscles in your face again, hold it for three to five seconds, and release. As you release the tension in the muscles, really let the tension leave your facial muscles. Continue to breathe as you feel these muscles become more relaxed.

Now, concentrate all your attention on your neck and shoulders, but allow your facial muscles to remain relaxed. Tense the muscles in your neck and shoulders by raising your shoulders up toward your earlobes. Tense all these muscles and hold it. Hold the tension for about three to five seconds and release the muscles. Notice the difference between the feelings of tension and relaxation. Tense the muscles in your neck and shoulders again. Hold it for three to five seconds, and release. As you release the tension in the muscles, really let the tension leave your neck and shoulders. Continue to breathe as you feel these muscles become more deeply relaxed.

Now concentrate all your attention on your arms, but allow your neck and shoulder muscles to remain relaxed.

Concentrate on the muscles in your arms and hands. Tense the muscles in your arms by bending your elbows upwards, and in your arms by making fists. Tense all these muscles and hold it. Hold the tension for about three to five seconds and release the muscles. Notice the difference between the feelings of tension and relaxation. Tense the muscles in your arms and hands again, hold it for three to five seconds, and release. As you release the tension in the muscles, really let the tension leave your face, neck and shoulders, and arms and hands. With each body part you are becoming more and more relaxed. Continue to breathe as you feel these muscles become more deeply relaxed.

Now concentrate all your attention on your torso, but allow the muscles in your arms to remain relaxed. Tense the muscles in your torso by standing up or sitting as straight as you can. Tense all these muscles and hold it. Hold the tension for about three to five seconds and release the muscles. Notice the difference between the feelings of tension and relaxation. Tense the muscles in your torso again, hold it for three to five seconds, and release. As you release the tension in the muscles, really let the tension leave your body. With each body part you are becoming more and more relaxed. Continue to breathe as you feel these muscles become more deeply relaxed.

Now concentrate all your attention on your legs and feet, but allow your body to remain relaxed. Tense the muscles in your legs by keeping them straight and in your feet by flexing them upwards. Tense all these muscles and hold it. Hold the tension for about three to five seconds and release the muscles. Notice the difference between the feelings of tension and relaxation. Tense the muscles in your legs and feet again, hold it for three to five seconds, and release. As you release the tension in the muscles, really let the tension leave your body. With each body part you are becoming more and more relaxed. Continue to breathe as you feel these muscles become more deeply relaxed.

You may choose to perform PMR on all of your body parts or not. After you have practiced this exercise several times, you will not need to keep practicing the tension part of the exercise, as you will be able to simply relax your muscles. Remember that practicing relaxation exercises is the key to success. *If you do these exercises only once or twice, and you don't see any results, it is because these exercises do not work if you do them only once or twice.* Regular practice is the key to maximizing the benefits you can obtain from relaxation exercises.

Guided Imagery

Guided imagery, or visualization, is a type of relaxation exercise in which you visualize a particular situation or image to decrease tension and increase feelings of relaxation. In guided imagery, you make use of all of your senses: sight, hearing, taste, touch, and smell. For example, many people visualize themselves at the beach. They relax when they imagine they are hearing the ocean, feeling the sand between their toes, smelling the salty air, feeling the sun on their face, etc.

You may wish to visualize yourself at the beach, in the mountains, at a family picnic, wherever it is that you feel most relaxed and at peace with yourself. Visualizing yourself in a situation where you feel peaceful and relaxed will assist you in decreasing any tension you may feel.

You can use visualizations as a way to cope with physical pain, as well. Patrick is a forty-one-year-old man with Crohn's disease who frequently gets abdominal pain and cramping. Whenever he feels pain in his stomach, he pictures Ezeriah, a red devilishlike creature whom he imagines lives in his stomach. When Patrick feels pain in his stomach, he visualizes Ezeriah having a temper tantrum. In his mind, he talks to Ezeriah, calms him down, and his pain gradually subsides. Patrick also says that he sometimes yells at Ezeriah, but when he does that, the devilish creature becomes even angrier, and Patrick's abdominal pain worsens. Patrick says that no matter how inconvenient Ezeriah's temper tantrums are, he must treat him with kindness and compassion. If not, his abdominal pain increases.

Sherry is a fifty-two-year-old woman who has lived with Crohn's disease for almost thirty years. When she gets abdominal pain, she pictures a balloon expanding in her stomach as her pain increases. The balloon gets bigger and bigger as the pain gets worse and worse. When Sherry can no longer stand the pain, she pops the imaginary balloon inside of her body, and she says the pain goes away.

These are some examples of how people with Crohn's disease cope with their physical pain. Not all of these examples will work for you; some will certainly work better than others. You may wish to make an audiotape of these exercises so that you can listen to the instructions while you practice. How you choose to help yourself relax is an individual decision. Regardless of your method of relaxation, it is essential to practice regularly. If relaxing for you means going to the movies, well, then, that's an activity: It is not a "relaxation technique" per se. But if going to the movies helps you to relax, do it.

Coping Strategies

There are many different ways you can cope with a situation. When you "cope" or deal with a certain situation or event, you may either increase or decrease the stress in your life. Relaxation techniques, like those described above, are ways to cope with pain and/or stress. As you have probably already guessed, coping can be very different for different people. You may know many people with Crohn's disease who handle situations very differently than you do. Just as everyone's disease process is different, and just as you are all unique individuals, you all have varying ways of living with Crohn's disease.

Coping with Crohn's disease may or may not be challenging for you. The disease may affect your life on a daily basis only when you are sick. Regardless of whether you are ill or not, you still have to cope with the fact that you have the disease. As the title of the book implies, dealing with this illness may involve a variety of challenges, both physical and emotional. Coping in an effective and productive manner can help you to adjust to your illness, regardless of whether it is active or quiescent, as well as help you in situations unrelated to your disease.

When you choose to cope with a problem in a way that makes you feel better about the situation, you are coping in a way that is successful and productive for you. There are two main ways of coping, or dealing with situations, people, and events. You can cope with a situation by changing your thoughts, or you can cope with it by changing your behaviors (Antoni and Schneiderman 1998; Antoni, Schneiderman, and Ironson 2000).

Problem-Focused Coping

When you cope with a situation by trying to fix the problem or the situation itself, you are coping in a "problem-focused" manner. Problem-focused coping involves trying to fix the problem or situation, rather than your thoughts and feelings about it. When you cope in a problem-focused manner, you think about the situation or difficulty, and problem-solve, or make decisions about how the situation can be altered, and then you set about implementing those decisions in a way that makes you feel better.

For instance, do you remember James, the accountant? His situation was described at the beginning of this chapter. He had a problem getting to work on time. He coped in a problem-focused way, by changing his behavior, not his thoughts or feelings about his situation. He didn't want to disclose his illness to his boss, so he altered his behavior to accommodate his disease in a way that relieved the stress of worrying whether he would get to work on time. Is that what you would do if you were James? Maybe, maybe not. For James it was a successful and productive method of coping, which is what matters. Just as not every type of relaxation technique will be right for you, how you choose to cope with situations is up to you. You will know that you've handled a situation successfully when the outcome is that you feel better about it.

Emotion-Focused Coping

When you deal with a situation by changing what you think, you also change your feelings or emotions about the situation. This type of coping is called "emotion-focused" coping (Antoni and Schneiderman 1998; Antoni, Schneiderman, and Ironson 2000). Instead of trying to change the situation, you try to change your thoughts and emotions about the situation. In this type of coping, you change your perceptions about the problem you are handling.

For instance, if you are nervous about an upcoming job interview, you might change your thoughts about the interview, without having to change your behavior while you are interviewed. If you say to yourself, "I will get a job eventually," that statement may change your perception about the interview. The contrary statement, "If I don't do well in this interview, I won't get any job at all," will undoubtedly produce anxiety about the interview and might even affect your behavior during the interview. So, it is usually a better idea for you to think positive thoughts than negative ones.

When coping with active Crohn's disease, your behavior, namely needing to use a rest room, may affect your perception of certain events. For example, Davis is a thirty-three-year-old man who was asked to be best man at a friend's wedding. He became extremely nervous about walking down the aisle and standing still during the wedding ceremony. He thought, "I can't do this. What if I need to go to the bathroom, and I can't hold it. What will I do?" He told his friend, the groom, about his fears, because he just didn't think that he would be able to perform the role of best man, and he didn't want to be embarrassed. His friend understood Davis' fears, and was helpful to him. After the two talked about it for a while, Davis was able to change his perception of the upcoming task. He thought to himself, "What's the big deal? If I need to use the rest room, I'll go and find one. If I had asthma, and needed to cough or sneeze during the ceremony, that wouldn't stop me from walking down the aisle. I'm not going to let Crohn's disease prevent me from doing that either."

Is it better to deal with a situation with problem-focused or emotion-focused coping? It depends on the situation. Sometimes it may be useful to use both problem-focused and emotion-focused coping behaviors. For example, Regina was very anxious about having a colonoscopy. So, she began to practice relaxation exercises some weeks before the procedure was scheduled, which helped her to diminish her tension. She was able to reduce her nervousness and thought to herself, "This won't be so bad. It won't be as overwhelming as I think it would." She also spoke to other patients who had recently had colonoscopes themselves.

The night before the operation was scheduled, when she drank the preparatory drink, she said that she pretended it was chocolate milk, and drank it quickly, thus changing her perception of the drink (even if she didn't change the actual taste), and she used visualization and guided imagery, as well. Regina illustrates the use of both problem-focused and emotion-focused coping. She was able to change both her behavior and her emotions before having her colonoscopy, so that when the procedure actually took place, her nervousness about the entire situation was considerably decreased.

The second half of this book will provide you with ways to handle emotionally difficult situations that arise as a consequence of having Crohn's disease, as well as information about social support and nutrition. As you continue reading, try to remember that how you cope with Crohn's disease is as individual as the disease itself. If something works for you, such as keeping a pain diary, doing a particular relaxation exercise, or using a specific way of coping, don't let anyone tell you otherwise. Keep your physician informed of all the situations, activities, and/or people that help you in dealing with your illness. It will help you to establish and maintain an alliance with your doctor against your disease. If you believe you can control your thoughts and your feelings in a way that you feel works for you, then you can.

PART II

Emotional Challenges

Chapter 6

In Search of
Your New Self

Whether or not your disease is active, Crohn's disease is a part of who you are. Acknowledging that you do have feelings about having this disease, regardless of what those feelings are, is an essential part of dealing with it from an emotional perspective. The twelve-step programs' famous Serenity Prayer states: "God grant me the ability to accept the things I cannot change, the ability to change the things I can, and the wisdom to know the difference." You may not be able to change the fact that you have Crohn's disease, but there are ways to increase your understanding of your illness and your feelings surrounding it.

The remainder of this book discusses ways to help you deal with the emotional challenges that living with Crohn's disease presents, such as understanding the emotional impact of the disease, telling other people that you have it, and forming and maintaining intimate relationships. It also discusses the reasons why a good social support system and proper nutrition are important to you as a person living with Crohn's disease.

Reciprocity Between Crohn's Disease and Your Emotions

Emotions are very powerful forces. They influence perceptions, thoughts, and behaviors. They can also influence you physically. Today, many people are studying "mind-body" interactions because during the past twenty years, a large amount of multidisciplinary research has led to the belief that the mind and body interact with each other in ways that can promote and/or hinder your health, physically and emotionally.

For example, think about what happens when you have a "tension" headache. Your head is in physical pain. When physical pain is felt, your emotions change. You may become irritable and cranky. When you have a headache, you probably don't want to be friendly or nice to others. You probably want to take two pills and just go to sleep. Once your physical symptoms cease, your mood and your demeanor change, and it is likely that you will become friendlier. Now, while headaches may vanish with pills, your Crohn's disease is always present, active or not. Hence, taking care of yourself emotionally and physically is important to your overall sense of well-being, regardless of your disease activity. You may already know that, at times, the physical symptoms of your disease can be difficult to handle. But you may not know that your emotional and psychological reactions to your illness may be equally as challenging.

How Emotions Influence Crohn's Disease

The impact of your emotions on your illness relates to how your emotions and feelings influence your overall sense of well-being. Your feelings in any given moment affect your thoughts and your behaviors, whether they concern Crohn's disease or not. Everyone has unique reactions to adverse events, and the range of emotional reactions one might experience to a given event is large. There are no right or wrong emotional responses. Emotions/feelings aren't right or wrong, they just are.

For example, when you become emotionally upset, you may stop eating, or become irritable, or withdrawn. You could be sad or angry. Sometimes, you may choose not to think about an upsetting event or situation at all, and proceed with the daily activities of your life as if everything were fine. You could also choose to handle upsetting situations with problem-focused and/or emotion-focused methods for coping, as discussed in chapter 5. The decisions that you make regarding difficult situations may be based on your feelings about those situations.

When you have Crohn's disease and you become upset, you may notice that your disease responds to your emotional state almost immediately. For instance, the number of times you need to use the bathroom may increase. Why? Because when you are emotionally upset, the physical part of your body most likely to be affected is your gut; thus, increased diarrhea or abdominal cramping, or constipation (if those are your symptoms) may result. Why would your emotions affect your gut? Because your gut is where you are most likely to be physically vulnerable. Don't misunderstand, your feelings *may* affect your disease process, they don't necessarily *have* to affect your disease process. You may become emotionally upset and not see any change in your symptoms. Generally speaking, it all depends on how your emotions affect you.

If emotions caused the disease, you would be able to cure it with happiness, joy, and pleasure. Unfortunately, it doesn't work that way. Happiness and pleasure in your life may help you to become more tolerant of periods of active disease, but pleasurable feelings don't cause the disease to go away. You can live a happy, loving, and successful life, and still have active Crohn's disease. You are more likely to have a greater tolerance for your disease activity when you are feeling happy with your life and yourself.

Conversely, when you feel sad, upset, angry, and stressed, your tolerance for your disease activity may decrease and you may feel increasingly unhappy with both your disease and yourself on a daily basis. In this manner, happiness will not cure your disease, but emotions like sadness, anger, and frustration definitely can affect it.

To provide you with better care and to maximize your overall health, studies have been conducted on psychological symptoms and the overall quality of life (Drossman, 1995, 1996; Garrett and Drossman, 1990; Ramchandani, Schindler, and Katz 1994). Nevertheless, despite all of the people afflicted with Crohn's disease and the amount of research conducted in this area, the relationship between psychological and physiological symptoms remains ambiguous (Trachter, Sellers, Katell, and Ishii 2000).

Drossman (1995; 1996) stated that the greater your psychological discomfort, the lower your pain tolerance is, and the more likely you are to seek health care. As previously stated, when you are emotionally upset, your tolerance for pain, diarrhea, and cramping may decrease. You may visit the doctor more often. The evidence suggests that better psychological functioning (e.g., overall life satisfaction) is associated with more adaptive coping with disease-related stress and the use of psychosocial factors like social support and self-control (Drossman 1996; Trachter, Sellers, Katell, and Ishii 2000).

How Crohn's Disease Influences Emotions

According to Olbrisch and Ziegler (1982) the disease process influences both your personality and your emotional status. Some researchers have suggested that as disease activity increases, both your physiological and psychological functioning deteriorate (Robertson, Jay, Diamond, and Edwards 1989; Drossman 1995). This should make sense to you. As you increasingly spend more time in the bathroom and increasingly experience greater physical discomfort, it wears on your psyche, whether you consciously recognize it or not. When you consistently don't feel physically well, it is understandable that your emotional state would become affected.

Appearances May Not Be Accurate

It can be emotionally difficult to deal with Crohn's disease for reasons other than the symptoms of active disease. Think about what you feel like when you have the flu. Do you feel upbeat and happy? Active Crohn's disease is much like a chronic flu, only you don't necessarily look sick. Have you ever felt physically awful and had someone tell you how wonderful you look? Have you ever heard, "I don't know how you feel, but you look wonderful!" when you've been feeling unwell for quite some time? How do statements like these affect you?

Pam, a thirty-three-year-old woman who has had Crohn's disease for ten years, said that she frequently hears comments like the one above, especially when she is feeling physically at her worst. She attributes the comments to the fact that when she is very ill, she loses weight and appears to be thinner than she usually looks. Pam reports that when people make such comments to her, she says thank you, but becomes frustrated because, "Just because I don't look sick, doesn't mean I don't feel sick."

Increasing your awareness of how you handle such situations will help you to understand how your feelings influence your thoughts and your behaviors. Pam illustrates the discrepancy between physical appearance and physical compromise. She doesn't feel well, but she looks wonderful. One of the many challenges of living with Crohn's is that you don't necessarily have to *look* sick in order to *be* sick.

Establishing Your Emotional Responses

Your awareness of how your emotions influence your thoughts and decision making (e.g., your behaviors) is important in ascertaining how your emotions and your disease interact with one another. You can more easily identify the influence of your emotions on your disease process if you understand how your emotions influence you. How can you do that? Ask yourself the following questions:

- Am I an emotional person? Are my emotions easily aroused?

- How do I express my feelings? When I express my feelings, how are they communicated?

- How do my feelings influence my thoughts? How do my feelings influence my behaviors?

First, answer these questions without Crohn's disease in your mind. Answer the questions for each of the emotions discussed in chapter 1, that is, denial, anger, depression, etc. Greater awareness of how you express depression, anger, fear, and anxiety will give you a greater understanding of yourself, regardless of your disease process. For the emotion of depression, for instance, you could ask yourself:

- How do I feel when I am sad? How do I express sadness? How do other people know that I am sad? How does sadness influence my thoughts and my actions?

Ask yourself each of these questions for the entire range of emotions that you may experience. Then, when you have answered them to your satisfaction, ask yourself these questions again, but this time add "about Crohn's disease" to each question.

- Am I emotional about Crohn's disease?

- How do I express my feelings about Crohn's disease? When I express my feelings about Crohn's disease, how are they communicated?

- How do my feelings about Crohn's disease influence my thoughts? How do my feelings about Crohn's disease influence my behaviors?

Are your responses to the second set of questions the same, or are they different? Once you have a greater understanding of how you express your feelings, and the role your feelings play in your thoughts and behaviors, you can apply that knowledge to your disease process. For instance, when do you notice that your physical symptoms are increasing? How do you feel when you notice the increase in your physical symptoms? Is there anything happening in your life that might be influencing your disease (e.g., relationship- or job-related stress)? If you find that you express your feelings about Crohn's disease differently than you express your feelings in general, consider talking to a professional about this discrepancy in your emotional responses.

Paying attention to when your physical symptoms increase can be very helpful to understanding when you are most vulnerable to active disease. It will also provide you with more information about your entire disease process, which you might consider sharing with your physician. This is part of having a collaborative relationship with your physician (see chapter 2).

For example, did you notice that your symptoms increased right after a major life change, such as relocating to a different home? Changing jobs or moving to a new home are major life changes. If you call your physician to talk about your increase in symptoms, telling the doctor that you've moved provides him/her with a more comprehensive picture of your disease activity and the situations and/or events that might have had some influence on your illness. Noticing when your symptoms increase and how you were feeling just prior to the increase will give you additional helpful information.

There is no strong conclusive and consistent research that states clearly that emotions are the cause of the disease, nor that the disease is the cause of certain emotions. It is, however, generally agreed that there is some kind of reciprocal relationship between your emotions and Crohn's disease. Furthermore, dealing with your emotions will be helpful to both your emotional state and physical well-being.

Stress and Crohn's Disease

Emotions are also influenced by the amount and type of stress in your life. Chronic illness itself is stressful, which will adversely affect your psyche (Casselith, Lusk, Strouse, Miller, et al. 1984; Drossman, 1995). Thus, just having Crohn's disease may be stressful for you, aside from the physical symptoms you may or may not experience.

The relationship between stress and the physical symptoms of people with both Crohn's disease and ulcerative colitis has been investigated (Duffy, Zielenzy, Marshall, Byers, et al. 1991; Garrett, Brantley, Jones, and McKnight 1991; Greene, Blanchard, and Wan 1994; McKegney, Gordon, and Levine 1970; North, Alpers, Helzer, et al. 1991). Although psychosocial factors (e.g., depression, anger, and anxiety) may not cause disease activity, psychosocial stressors (e.g., relationships, work, etc.) may influence disease activity (Talal and Drossman 1995; Drossman 1996). The identification and clarification of those activities and situations that "stress you out" would be helpful to both your physical and emotional well-being, as it would allow you to handle such situations in a manner that optimizes your overall well-being and quality of life, as opposed to hindering it.

The Literature Says . . .

Studies also have examined the relationship between stress and disease activity specifically in individuals with Crohn's disease. In a study conducted by Sessions, Raft, and Tate (1978) that evaluated the relationship between stress, depression, anxiety, and disease activity among those with Crohn's disease, the findings indicated that life stress, depression, and anxiety were not clearly related to the severity of the disease. In a later study Garrett, Brantley, Jones, and McKnight (1991) monitored daily stress and symptoms of Crohn's disease for twenty-eight days. In this study, a relationship between daily stress and severity of symptoms was established. The findings of this study supported the work of other researchers in the field (Drossman 1995; Fullwood and Drossman 1995; Garrett, Brantley, Jones, and McKnight 1991).

These contradictory findings in the scientific literature illustrate the difficulty in establishing a clear and consistent relationship between stress and Crohn's disease. As a result, it is difficult to know with any certainty whether stress exacerbates disease symptoms or disease symptoms exacerbate stress. The question is similar to "Which came first? The chicken or the egg?" A thorough review of the literature would find evidence for both positions. Nevertheless, if you can identify stressful situations quickly and manage your stress effectively, you are better able to manage the effects of your disease.

What Is Stress?

Stress, according to Webster, is mental or physical tension or strain. Identifying stressful situations and/or events is helpful so that you can manage those kinds of situations in a way that optimizes your physical and emotional health. There are many ways stress can affect you, physically, emotionally, cognitively, and behaviorally. Your body does have physical responses to stress, whether you have noticed it or not. But you're the one who has to figure out how it manifests itself in you.

You may experience a variety of the physical effects of stress. When you are under stress, you may find that you need to go to the bathroom more often. You may find that your heart races, or your muscles tighten. Perhaps you perspire. Taking notice of how your body responds to stress will also help you with the relaxation exercises discussed in chapter 5. Notice which parts of your body hold tension, and focus on those body parts when you're practicing the relaxation exercises (e.g., your neck, shoulders, etc.).

Stress also influences your feelings and thoughts. When you are in a stressful situation, you may become more irritable or overly sensitive. You may have less tolerance and patience for people and situations. Your thoughts may become affected as well. Your thought processes might be different than they would otherwise be. In stressful situations, you may experience both emotional and cognitive responses/reactions. Consequently, your behavior may be different when you are under stress than it might be otherwise.

For example, your appetite and sleep habits may change. You may have less energy to do the tasks you normally do. As stated throughout the first half of the book, your feelings and thoughts affect your behavior. It is up to you to identify how stress affects you.

Identifying Stressful Situations

A clear understanding of those situations and events that stress you out is needed before you can ascertain your emotional and physical responses to those situations. Ask yourself the following questions:

1. What situations cause you stress?

2. How do you know that you are under stress?

3. Do you behave differently when under stress (i.e., do you smoke, drink, cry, eat, sleep more, etc.)?

4. How does your body respond to stress (more bathroom use, more abdominal pain, more headaches, etc.)?

5. What types of feelings do you have when under stress?

6. What types of thoughts do you have when under stress?

7. What happens to your disease when you are under stress? Are your symptoms affected? If so, how?

The answers to these questions will help you to manage stressful situations as they arise, because when you are aware of your thoughts and feelings, you will be more able to control them and, consequently, more able to control your behaviors in an effective manner.

The relationship between stress and symptom exacerbation in individuals with both Crohn's disease and ulcerative colitis requires further clarification (Eysselein 2000). Schwarz and Blanchard (1990) reported "Obviously, the effects of psychosocial stressors on either the onset or the exacerbation of IBD [inflammatory bowel disease] are far from being clearly understood. More well-controlled studies are needed to help clarify this aspect of these diseases" (101).

You may not know for certain whether stress exacerbates your disease, or whether your disease exacerbates your stress level. Common sense suggests that it is likely to be a combination of both and, thus, a reciprocal cycle. How do you break the cycle? Identifying stressful situations is only a part of managing Crohn's disease effectively. Your attitude and your expectations, as well as how you communicate them, can help you to alleviate stress.

Attitude

Your attitude and your expectations can help you to decrease your stress level. Your attitude can either assist or hinder your daily activities. Your *attitude* refers to your opinion or mental state of being that influences your behavior. It modulates the way you incorporate Crohn's disease into your life. Your attitude can be of great assistance to you throughout your life because it can help you when you feel most upset. Your attitude toward relationships, work, *and your disease* influences your feelings and your thoughts and, consequently, how you choose to handle stressful situations when they arise.

Remember, perception is everything. If your perception of yourself is positive, it will affect everything you do. People take their lead from you. If you have a positive attitude, those around you will react to you in a positive way, especially when it comes to your disease. For instance, if you believe that Crohn's disease is only as significant as your eye or hair color, that's how significant it will be to you, and to others, as well. What about the fact that you are having diarrhea three times a day? Well, that is a symptom of your disease; it is not who you are as a person. If you believe that you are your disease, you will find it more difficult to treat the disease as only a part of your life. For some, there may be times when Crohn's disease will feel as though it is your whole life, because you may become very ill. It is at those times especially, that your attitude is most critical. During those hard times, try to remember that Crohn's disease will not be your whole life forever; it will eventually quiet down.

The Power of Positivity

Tony is a thirty-six-year-old who has had Crohn's disease since he was fourteen. He was sick for most of his teenage years. His last active period of disease occurred at the age of nineteen, when he underwent a resection. For two and a half consecutive years prior to his surgery, he was very ill. He was in and out of the hospital several times, required home schooling for a while, and, finally, underwent a resection. Throughout that period of his life, Tony remained upbeat and positive. Although there were times when he became frustrated and upset with his situation, those occasions were the exceptions, not the rule. He did say that it had been very difficult for him at times; he had become angry and yelled at his family and friends, as well as the hospital staff. But he also tried to remain hopeful about his future, and maintain his confidence that one day he would feel better.

Currently, Tony feels well, is married, and has a two-year-old daughter. He smiles and laughs often, makes jokes about his disease, and believes that, with a positive attitude, anything in life is possible. He has not had active disease since the time of his surgery, seventeen years ago. Although he realizes that the disease may become active again, he feels that he will have the ability to handle it when, or if, that time arrives.

Your attitude says much about who you are as an individual. Tony did not, and does not relinquish his ability to hope for good physical health, to anyone. His attitude helped him through difficult times with Crohn's disease, and it is very likely that it has assisted him in other areas of his life, too. He was able to allow himself to feel hurt, frustrated, angry, and disappointed, but not so much so that those emotions consumed him or stopped him from pursuing his life goals. Tony remained true to his dreams, his hopes, and his aspirations; his attitude assisted him in that process.

Your perception of yourself influences other people's perceptions of you. If you present yourself in a manner that is positive, others are more likely to perceive you as a "positive person." If you perceive yourself in a negative manner, others are likely to agree with you. Other people take their lead from you.

Shame Related to Bodily Functions

Because Crohn's disease is a disease that deals with diarrhea, burping, gas, and quite frankly, shit, shame is an emotion that may arise, but it is a feeling that you may not discuss. Talking about feces, unless you are talking to a doctor, is a taboo. Funny smells and odors are rarely discussed in "polite" society. If you've ever had an accident, smelled up a public bathroom, or passed gas in an elevator, shame and/or embarrassment are not unfamiliar to you. However, you are not your disease. You are not shameful, neither is your behavior.

If someone with cancer, who was receiving chemotherapy, suddenly vomited in public, would you consider such behavior shameful or embarrassing? If someone with asthma had an asthma attack at a party, and started to wheeze, sneeze, and cough uncontrollably, would that be considered shameful and/or embarrassing? Diarrhea, burping, or passing gas caused by a disease is not any different.

Although you may think this makes sense to you, try to remember how you felt when situations like these occurred. Were you comfortable or uncomfortable? What were you feeling when you knew you weren't going to make it to the bathroom? What did you think? What did you feel? How did you behave? What does thinking about these situations now bring up for you? If you are fortunate enough never to have had an accident like this, how does it make you feel to think that you might loose control of your bowels in public one day?

Why does knowing in advance what your emotional reactions to such situations would be help? It helps because self-awareness in situations like these empowers you. Self-awareness gives you the ability to control your thoughts, your feelings, and your behaviors. It helps you to communicate to those around you in a way that makes it easier to be comfortable with yourself. If you can identify and explain to yourself what it is that increases your comfort level in situations like those described above, you will find it easier to communicate it to others. Only you can answer these questions. Only you know what you think, how you feel, and how you have behaved in such situations, or how you would behave if situations should arise. The faster you find answers to these questions, the greater your ability to manage your life effectively and productively will be.

Sizing Up Shame

Shari is a twenty-year-old undergraduate who was recently diagnosed with Crohn's disease. She was placed on medication due to her frequent diarrhea, abdominal cramping, and low-grade fever. Shari lives in a college dormitory with the other coeds. As in many college dormitories, the bathrooms are located down the hallway and shared amongst the people living on the floor. Shari hasn't told her roommate or her other friends about her diagnosis. She wakes up periodically in the middle of the night to use the rest room; and she tries to use the bathroom when no one else is around for maximum privacy.

Shari states that she is quite self-conscious about using "bath-rooms in public." She says that she gets embarrassed by the odor, especially if the people whom she lives with are also using the facilities. Over several weeks, Shari became increasingly nervous and anxious, constantly worried that not only would she have an accident, but that someone would "find out."

Such self-consciousness is not uncommon. Shari's concern about other people "finding out" is also noteworthy. What if someone did find out? What if she told the senior resident on the hall? What if she had asked for help to decrease her anxiety? How is carrying such a burden of nervous, anxious thoughts and feelings around helpful? Perhaps you have experienced a similar situation. How did you handle it? Did you think, feel, and behave similarly? Why or why not? How would you handle a similar situation today? How you handle situations like these, how you think about them, and how you feel about them influences your perceptions of yourself and your body.

Self-Image and Body Image

Defecation is a natural physical function; however, on a constant basis, the symptoms of Crohn's disease may engender feelings of shame about defecation, which may decrease both self-image and body image. Spending a majority of your time during the day on a toilet may not promote a healthy body image or positive feelings regarding your genitalia. The unreliability of the disease process and the fear of unexpected symptoms may permeate your self-esteem and your psyche in an insidious manner. You may not even realize it is happening.

For instance, having to use a bathroom urgently and "having an accident" as an adult may influence your self-confidence. After all, you are taught to "control" your bowels as a young child. What does it mean to you to lack "control" as an adult? Consider this question as you continue to read this book. Consider the role "control" plays in your life.

Fears of being viewed as "sick" might also affect your self-image and erode your sense of self. You may fear being thought of as deficient in some way. Perhaps that may be why some people with Crohn's disease don't discuss their disease openly. Like Shari, perhaps you have a fear of being "found out." Again, only you know how you feel about disclosure. See chapter 7 for a discussion about disclosure.

Body Image and Behaviors

Aaron is a single nineteen-year-old male who was diagnosed with Crohn's disease at the age of seventeen. Throughout his undergraduate education, his disease was treated with medication therapy. In the last six months, the medications were unable to control his disease, and surgery was recommended. Aaron reported feeling "Sick of being sick. I just want to feel okay and do the things that my friends do." Aaron is in a fraternity and frequently attends fraternity parties with his peers. However, he has not told anyone outside of his immediate family that he has Crohn's. He recently sought psychotherapy because of an incident that occurred at a fraternity party and because of his anxiety about his upcoming operation.

Aaron had attended a fraternity party where he drank heavily, despite the fact that alcohol exacerbates his diarrhea. Due to the large number of people at the party, he was forced to wait on line to use the rest room. Although he tried, he couldn't restrain himself and, evidently, he defecated in his clothing in the hallway of the fraternity house. Some of the other drunken coeds noticed and proceeded to ostracize him, both for the odor and his inability "to control himself." Aaron stated, "I'm so embarrassed and ashamed. No one will ever date me now."

This case vignette illustrates the difficulties that may arise if you are a young adult with Crohn's disease. It also demonstrates the insidious impact the disease may have on body image, sexuality, and interpersonal relationships. Perhaps Aaron should not have been drinking, and perhaps the coeds should not have ostracized him for his "accident." Nonetheless, the interaction cannot be discounted, especially in regard to its influence on both Aaron's body image and sexual image.

Aaron has stated many times that he no longer feels "attractive." Moreover, he is concerned that the scar from the upcoming operation will further "wreck his body." Clearly, Aaron's perceives his body as "damaged." His poor body image and perceived lack of attractiveness promote his secrecy with regard to his disease. He reported, "If people don't know, they won't think differently of me." Clearly, your expectations of yourself influence how you interact and communicate with those around you.

Realistic Expectations

Expectations are those goals, actions, behaviors that you set for yourself and others. Your expectations of yourself may be similar to or different from your expectations of others. When your expectations of yourself are realistic, you accomplish those tasks you've decided to perform, regardless of whether they pertain to your personal or professional life, or not.

When your expectations are unrealistic, you may not accomplish those tasks that you set out to perform. Unrealistic expectations of yourself may lead to frustration, disappointment, and emotional upset. In this manner, your expectations of yourself influence your attitude. For example, if you set out to achieve certain goals in an unrealistic time frame, your ability to complete those tasks is hindered by time constraints. An inability to achieve your expectations can have an adverse impact on the way you approach the tasks at hand. Your expectations of yourself may affect the people around you, as well.

There are several ways that your expectations can have an impact on those around you. When you meet your expectations of yourself, that can lead to more positive feelings about yourself and, consequently, have a more positive effect on those around you. Why? Because your attitude changes, as do your thoughts and feelings surrounding the tasks, or the expectations of yourself that remain. The following chart illustrates the process:

Remember James? His situation was discussed in chapter 5. He was the individual who set his alarm clock earlier in the morning so he could arrive at work on time without having to tell his boss about his disease. His expectations of himself were such that he wanted to be on time for work, yet the disease prevented him from doing so, unless he altered his schedule. James' boss' expectation that James should arrive at work promptly was also realistic. Have you ever heard the phrase "There's more than one way to skin a cat"? Well, that means that you always have options available to you. Your expectations of yourself and other people's expectations of you can and do change, especially when you are physically compromised because of active Crohn's disease. Communicating realistic expectations to those around you, especially when you are experiencing an active disease can help you during your daily routine.

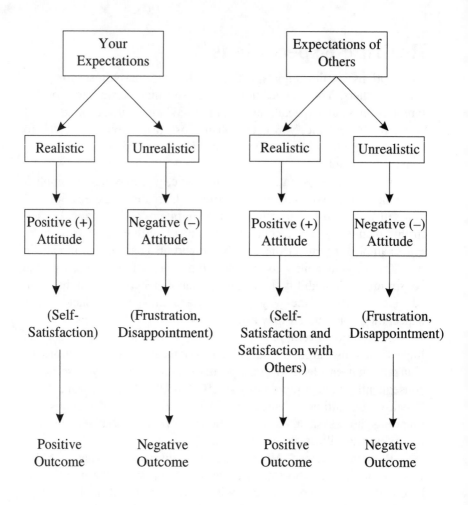

Your Expectations		Expectations of Others	
Realistic	Unrealistic	Realistic	Unrealistic
Positive (+) Attitude	Negative (–) Attitude	Positive (+) Attitude	Negative (–) Attitude
(Self-Satisfaction)	(Frustration, Disappointment)	(Self-Satisfaction and Satisfaction with Others)	(Frustration, Disappointment)
Positive Outcome	Negative Outcome	Positive Outcome	Negative Outcome

Communication

In addition to your attitude and your expectations, the manner in which you communicate is also important. The way in which you express your thoughts and feelings helps others to understand your disease and how you are choosing to deal with it. How you choose to express yourself is as important as what you choose to communicate. Remember communication is accomplished in two ways: nonverbal and verbal.

Nonverbal Communication

Nonverbal communication includes facial expressions, body posture, and eye contact. It also includes intonation, volume, and speed of your speech. Nonverbal communication can be very powerful. You may know people who speak volumes via their facial expressions, without ever having to say a word. Your nonverbal communication may be representative of how you're feeling. A smile, for instance, is usually interpreted as happiness; a frown as sadness. Raised eyebrows, the way you stand, how you position your body are all different forms of communication. Paying attention to your nonverbal mannerisms will help you to communicate your thoughts and feelings accurately and effectively.

For example, how often do you wince when you feel a stomach pain or cramp? Do you control your desire to clutch your stomach when it hurts you? If you are not aware of your nonverbal habits of communicating, you may be more likely to communicate in ways that are not helpful to you. Sometimes, your nonverbal behaviors may communicate an idea that you really don't mean to say. For example, when you have a conversation with your boss and you physically feel an abdominal pain, your nonverbal behaviors may be quite different from your verbal behavior. You might respond verbally in a very upbeat way to your boss, while making a face and clutching your stomach in an anxious way. Thus, you might be contradicting your upbeat message with the anxiety you feel, and that could send your boss a mixed message.

Verbal Communication

Verbal communication refers to how thoughts and feelings are expressed in words. You have control over what you say and how you say it. When you speak about Crohn's disease, how you speak is as important as what you say. The intonation and inflection of your voice, as well as your facial expressions, communicate your feelings about the disease as much as the content of your speech. For instance, if you were to tell a friend that you had Crohn's disease, and it wasn't troublesome to you, but you became tearful while you were speaking, your nonverbal communication might speak louder than your actual words.

Sometimes, it can be difficult to communicate verbally what you think and feel about your disease. Perhaps you don't like to speak about your disease at all. When you don't speak about your disease with others, or share your thoughts and feelings about the disease, what happens to those thoughts and feelings?

Perhaps you have inactive disease, and your disease doesn't affect you or your life (lucky you). In this context, your disease wouldn't necessarily require thought or discussion because it would have no impact on your daily functioning; however, understanding how you feel and think about your disease remains a goal that would be helpful to you.

For those of you with active disease who are experiencing physical symptoms, identifying and explaining your thoughts and feelings might be difficult. You may not want to talk about it: After all, you've got to live with it. Why discuss it, too? How do you explain what Crohn's disease is accurately and effectively, if most people you know aren't familiar with the disease, much less what your thoughts and feelings about it are? After all, Crohn's disease isn't like cancer, or diabetes, illnesses that people are quite familiar with and about which they have all sorts of information. Chapter 7 deals with how, when, why, and in which situations disclosure is appropriate. Identifying how (and if) you communicate your thoughts and feelings about your disease, especially when you are ill, may provide you with additional support, both physical and emotional, during your periods of active disease. Understanding how you communicate with regard to your disease and your symptoms increases your understanding of your own attitudes and expectations of yourself and others.

Hopefully, you will have a greater understanding of the role of stress in your entire disease process, as well as how you handle stressful situations. Using the coping methods described in chapter 5 will assist you in dealing with stressful situations. Try to remember there is no one correct way to handle stress, there is simply a way that will work best for you. Increasing your self-awareness with regard to your emotional reactions, attitudes, expectations, and communication habits will be of use to you throughout your life in various situations, not just with respect to your Crohn's disease.

Chapter 7

To Tell or
Not to Tell

Chapter 6 provided you with an increased understanding about the role of your emotions and stress in the disease process, as well as how your reactions, attitudes, and expectations may influence you as a person living with Crohn's disease. Identifying and recognizing your beliefs and ideas about your disease promotes your ability to communicate to others. This chapter concentrates on the who, when, why, and how of disclosure. Sometimes it is appropriate and necessary to disclose, sometimes it is not.

Perhaps some of what you read will be familiar to you. Maybe you don't need to say anything at all because your disease is inactive, and it is not affecting your life. Take in what you read merely as suggestions to help you adjust to your illness. Whether your disease is active or not, it is a part of who you are. Telling other people that you have the disease and informing them of how they can help you will be of assistance to you if and when you are physically compromised (e.g., sick).

Dispelling the Myths

Before you start to tell other people about your disease and how it might be affecting you, you should have a clear understanding of how you're going to go about presenting the information. People will ask you questions about your disease. The greater your understanding of what your disease means to you, the more able you will be to answer their questions. There are certain facts you can tell to people about Crohn's disease immediately that will increase their understanding. It is very likely you already know some of these facts, but a review may be in order.

Fast Facts

1. Crohn's disease isn't fatal. It is treatable and controllable with proper medical treatment.

2. Crohn's disease isn't curable. Ulcerative colitis may be cured through surgery. Crohn's disease is treatable and controllable with proper medical care.

3. Crohn's disease isn't a "Jewish disease." Crohn's disease doesn't discriminate; it can, and does, affect all people, regardless of race, religion, nationality, sex, or sexual orientation.

4. Crohn's disease isn't caused by stress. Stress may exacerbate your symptoms, but it doesn't cause the disease.

5. At this time, the cause of Crohn's disease is unknown. Researchers and scientists are trying to find out what causes it, but no one can say for certain, yet.

6. Crohn's disease is a physical disease; it is not psychosomatic. You did not cause your disease by way of your psychological state.

7. Crohn's disease is not caused by eating certain foods. Food does not cause the disease.

If you incorporate statements such as those above into your explanation of the disease, it will help others to understand it, and will circumvent some questions that might arise. Many people know about the disease only if they know someone who has it. Therefore, the information people receive from you may be the only information they have about it, unless they choose to read about it on their own, or hear about it from someone else. Consequently, how and what you say will influence others' perception of the disease. However, before the "how" and "what" aspects of disclosure can be discussed, you must first identify the "whom."

Disclosure: Whom to Tell

Whom you choose to impart knowledge of your disease to might be anyone and everyone. Part of being able to control the influence of the disease on your life includes being able to share that aspect of yourself with others, regardless of who they are. Providing information about your disease gives people a greater understanding of you, your life, and how you choose to live it.

Family

Your family, the people who love you most in the world, may include parents, grandparents, spouses, siblings, children, aunts, uncles, nieces and nephews, and cousins. Depending on the nature of your relationships with your family members, there are those with whom you will choose to share your experiences and those you won't. Your family, however you choose to define the people that comprise it, are the people who love and care about you. They want the best for you and wish for your happiness and good health.

When you first find out that you have Crohn's disease, you may choose to have one of your family members go with you when you visit your doctor. It is helpful to have someone with you when you first hear about your disease because that person will hear what the physician says to you, and then can act as a reality check for you after your visit, if need be. Also, you are less likely to forget what the doctor says about your disease, and more likely to remember questions you want to ask, if someone else is with you. This doesn't mean that you must have someone with you every time you go to the doctor but, initially, you certainly may find it helpful. In this manner, there will be at least one other person who knows about your disease without you having to say anything directly. But what about your other family members?

Think about what it would be like for you to hear that someone you love is sick. Maybe you'd be concerned. Maybe you'd worry. Maybe you'd want to know if there was anything you could do to help the family member feel better. What would it be like for you to know that someone you love is sick, and there is nothing you could do about it, and nothing that you can do to make that person feel better?

When you tell your family about your disease and how you are feeling, it will be helpful to them to know what is helpful for you. Give them the facts about the disease, an overview, as it were, first. Then give them the facts about *your* disease. State how you are being treated (i.e., medications, procedures needed, etc.) and what was recommended for the future. Initially, you may not know how family members can assist you, and that's okay. Inform the people who love you that when you figure it out, you'll let them know.

When to Let Your Family Know

When you share your diagnosis with your family may depend on how sick you are feeling. For instance, if you are diagnosed with the disease, take medication, and then feel better, it may be necessary to share the information only with the people with whom you live. If you become quite ill, you may feel the need to tell other family members what's happening to you, to make your life easier.

For instance, if you are not feeling well and can't eat very much, the change in your eating patterns may become noticeable to those around you. Perhaps family members will comment on the amount of food you've eaten, or the amount of weight that you have either gained or lost. Explaining why your eating habits have changed will give your family a better understanding of your behavior. You wouldn't want your family to think that you don't like food that they've prepared. But if you explain that you don't want to exacerbate your bowel, surely that would soothe any hurt feelings that might arise.

Some of you may tell family about your disease as new situations arise, and some of you may choose to pick a date and just tell them. When you tell family members, you should expect that questions will be asked. For some questions, you may know the answers, for others you won't. That's okay. Another reason that you might want to tell your family about your illness is that they may be of assistance to you. Perhaps they will give you some new perspectives and help you to perceive the whole situation differently. Perhaps telling them will make your interactions with them easier for you when you're not feeling well.

When the Family Knows

Holly is a twenty-seven-year-old woman who has had Crohn's disease for eight years. Her disease activity has waxed and waned over the eight-year span. She has been on and off a variety of medications, as well. Recently, she was experiencing some anxiety about an upcoming Thanksgiving dinner with her family. Both her immediate family (spouse, parents, and siblings) and her extended family (aunts, uncles, grandparents, etc.) knew of her Crohn's disease. Holly had explained that she could tolerate some foods, and not others. Over the years she has learned which foods cause her symptoms to increase.

For several weeks prior to Thanksgiving her disease had been bothersome to her. Yet again, she was experiencing active disease and was taking medication for it. Although she was looking forward to seeing her relatives, she was not looking forward to the questions that were bound to be asked. "How is she feeling?" "How is she doing?" "Is she feeling better?" "Is she not eating X and Y because X and Y make her sick?" "What kind of food could be prepared for her, so that she could eat more?" To add insult to injury, Thanksgiving was usually one of her favorite meals, and she knew she'd be able to eat only the turkey and the potatoes. She wanted to be able to eat the sweet potato pie, the vegetable dishes, the cranberry sauce and all the other good foods her family prepared; and she was feeling sad because she knew that she could not do so, without making herself sicker.

Holly was frustrated with her disease. She was sick of feeling sick. She didn't want to have to explain her behavior to anyone or to answer anybody's questions. She went to the Thanksgiving dinner with a heavy heart. Although she was thankful for her family and the people in her life, she didn't feel well. She wanted to be pleasant and joyful, but she was physically exhausted. Throughout the meal she was quiet, she answered her family's questions with "Fine, thank you for asking." Holly had all she could do to handle her physical symptoms; she didn't feel up to explaining them. Hence, she was polite and loving but not forthcoming about the state of her physical symptoms.

Sometimes, when your family knows about your disease, you may feel that you must provide explanations for your behavior. Maybe you do provide explanations. Nonetheless, if you feel that you are not prepared to answer any question posed to you, it's okay to say, "I appreciate your concern, but I really don't know how to answer that. When I do, I'll let you know."

You've acknowledged the concern that has been expressed, responded to the question, and not had to answer a question you might have been asking yourself. If you find certain questions intrusive, it is okay to say, "I appreciate your concern, but I don't really want to talk about it right now," or "I would rather not answer that question." You want to encourage comfort and ease. Answering questions that make you feel uncomfortable will increase your stress level, and not help you feel better.

Friends

There are many different types of friendships. You may have some friends with whom you wish to talk about your disease, and you may have friends you don't want to know. Depending on the friend and the context of your friendship you may choose not to say anything at all. You decide who knows about your disease. You can control with whom you choose to share facts about yourself. You may have friends who have Crohn's disease, you may not. A friend doesn't have to have Crohn's to offer you support, encouragement, and assistance.

The Power of Friendship

Cameron is a twenty-two-year-old man who has had Crohn's disease for a few years. For the most part, his disease is controlled with medication. On occasion he gets sharp, unexpected abdominal pain. He frequently socializes on the weekends with friends, and he likes to go dancing at local clubs. He has told most of his friends that he has Crohn's disease.

Cameron states that he tells the people he socializes with so that he feels more comfortable and less self-conscious. For example, when they all go out together, and he disappears into the bathroom for fifteen to twenty minutes at a time, he doesn't have to explain his disappearance.

Additionally, sometimes when he gets those unexpected cramps, it becomes difficult for him to concentrate on conversations. He reports that he sometimes winces in pain, but doesn't say that his stomach hurts. Sometimes when he doesn't admit to his discomfort, his friends will ask, "Do you not like what is being said or are you just in pain?" (Note the nonverbal message communicated by his wincing.) He reported that one time a group of his friends and he were coming out of a bar and one of them turned and asked him, "Do you have to go to the bathroom?" Cameron said he just sat down right where he was standing, and said, "No, I can tell when I need a bathroom; right now, I just need to sit down." So he sat down for a short time. His friends waited for him, and several minutes later everyone left.

Cameron's example demonstrates how your friends can be of help to you just by *knowing* what's happening. It wasn't a big deal to his friends to wait a few minutes before they left the club. They wanted Cameron to feel well and were willing to accommodate him. Cameron also communicated his needs clearly; he was able to tell his friends what he required in the moment to feel okay, and then did so. Although this isn't always possible in all social situations, certainly among your friends, it may be possible.

You may have friends who have Crohn's disease. Having other people around you who live with similar circumstances may also be a source of support and comfort. Sharing your ideas, your feelings, and your thoughts with someone who has had similar experiences may provide you with different ways of doing things or interacting with people or sharing your disease with others. See chapter 9 for a discussion that focuses specifically on social support.

When to Let Friends Know

The exact time to tell your friends about your disease varies, depending on the types of friendships you have with them. Telling your friend(s) about your illness should be as comfortable for you as talking about your family, your occupation, or the traffic on the highway. You're not making an announcement; you're sharing a part of your life with another person. You may choose not to discuss your disease with your friends, and that is your decision to make based on your own comfort level. Be aware, however, that for those of you with active disease, not sharing information about the disease process may have adverse effects on a friendship.

Rebecca is a thirty-four-year-old married woman who has had Crohn's disease for sixteen years. Her disease activity has flared over the years, and she underwent a resection at the age of twenty-eight. Her family is well informed about her disease, as are some of her friends. One day, Rebecca made dinner plans for herself and her husband with Carmen and Jeff, a couple with whom she recently had become friendly. The two couples were supposed to dine together one evening on the weekend. Due to Rebecca's disease activity, Rebecca had to cancel the dinner plans. She told Carmen that she "didn't feel up to it."

The two women rescheduled the dinner for the following week. The second time Rebecca cancelled, Carmen asked if she had been to her doctor. Rebecca thanked Carmen for her concern, and explained what was happening. It was at that moment that Rebecca disclosed the fact that she had active Crohn's disease, which was why she had cancelled twice at the last minute. Rebecca didn't want Carmen to take her two dinner cancellations personally, and she also didn't want her disease to affect their friendship, so disclosure at that point seemed like a good idea.

Coworkers and Acquaintances

Your coworkers include all the people with whom you work. You may spend a great deal of your time with your coworkers, or you may not. If they aren't involved in your life on a personal level, it is not necessary to tell associates or acquaintances in your workplace. Associates, colleagues, acquaintances, and neighbors are those with whom you may interact frequently, but only for certain distinct purposes. Talking about Crohn's disease simply may not be appropriate. It is not a topic that should be hidden or concealed either. For instance, if in the context of a conversation, the topic of Crohn's disease is brought up, you might choose to disclose information about your own disease. Typically, it is not necessary to make your disease a topic of conversation among people who don't know you very well.

When to Let Acquaintances Know

Sometimes, telling acquaintances and/or coworkers may be necessary. Why? You might need time off from work to have a procedure, for example, and it could require some rescheduling or reallocating of job responsibilities. The disease in your body may prevent you from fulfilling an immediate obligation or task, and you might need a coworker to drive you somewhere or a neighbor to feed your cat. Sometimes, you may have no choice but to tell people.

Whether it is your family, your friends, and/or your acquaintances, sharing your illness is most appropriate when you are comfortable doing so. Again, so much about this disease is individual, where it is in your body, how it manifests itself in you physically, how you handle the physical challenges that present themselves, and the people with whom you choose to share your disease.

Disclosure: Who Needs to Know

Clearly, the medical and health professionals who treat you need to know. The significant other(s) in your life also have a need to know about your disease. The medical and health professionals must know what's going on with your disease to help you feel better. As discussed in chapter 2, establishing and maintaining a collaborative relationship with your physician is essential to treating your disease properly. Your significant other, whether your spouse, live-in lover, or whomever you are involved with in an intimate and loving relationship needs to know because the disease is a part of who you are. Your significant other needs to love all of you, including the parts of you with Crohn's disease.

Medical/Health Professionals

Medical/health professionals are those people who hold medical and health-related jobs. They may include, but are not limited to, physicians, nurses, dentists, nutritionists, radiologists, psychologists, and X-ray technicians. Medical and health professionals may and typically do possess basic knowledge about Crohn's disease. Consequently, simply stating that you have Crohn's disease may be enough information for the person with whom you're dealing because s/he will know what it is, although sometimes you will be asked specific questions about your disease. Remember, the more information medical and health professionals have about your disease, the better able they are to assist you.

Significant Others: Partners

Significant others, those people with whom you share your life, need to know about your disease. Significant other refers to the person with whom you're intimately and emotionally involved. Your significant other needs to know about your disease, and any and all feelings and beliefs that you have about it. Why? Presumably, you love and care about each other. If your significant other was the one with the illness, wouldn't you want him/her to share their feelings and thoughts with you? Wouldn't you want to know about what they were going through?

Committed Relationships

When you're married or involved in a committed relationship and you find out that you have Crohn's, it is quite different from when you are single and dating and you find out you've got Crohn's disease. Disclosure about your disease (how and what to say) to someone you are dating is different from telling a spouse or partner in the context of a committed relationship. See chapter 8 for a discussion of the impact that Crohn's disease may have on partnerships and dating relationships. In this chapter, relationships are discussed only with regard to disclosure.

Telling a spouse or partner about your disease is necessary to maintain the intimacy and trust that you have formed with your partner. It is not uncommon for partners/spouses to attend physician appointments together. When your spouse/partner goes with you to the physician, you don't have to repeat what the physician has said to you later in the day, because your partner was there and heard everything that you heard. However, your partner may not always be available to go with you. When that is the case, you will have to tell your partner what you and your physician have discussed. In the context of a committed relationship, disclosure in and of itself may not be an issue. However, your feelings about having the disease and your need to communicate those feelings to your partner might be. Again, see chapter 8 for a discussion of the impact of the disease on relationships.

Significant Others: Singles

Disclosure in the context of dating is an entirely different matter. For example, at what point do you tell someone you're dating that you've got a chronic illness? Much less one that makes you go to the bathroom frequently? What do you say? Some of you may choose to tell someone you are dating right away, some of you may date someone for six months before you feel ready to talk about your disease. Much of what you say and how you say it, depends on your disease, how you are feeling physically, and your own degree of comfort with it.

The more comfortable you are with yourself and your disease, the easier it will be to talk about it with other people, especially those you are dating. Why? When you're comfortable with yourself and your disease, talking about your disease isn't a big deal. Again, when you choose to share your disease with someone depends on when it is most comfortable for you to do so.

Early versus Late Disclosure

Rick is twenty-nine and has had Crohn's disease for six years. He tells the people he dates fairly early on in their dating relationship because he wants people to know quickly. He figures that he can "weed out" people by telling them early on in the relationship. On a date, Rick works the subject of Crohn's into the conversation, although he doesn't make an announcement. Rick feels that he wants to know right away whether someone can handle the possibility of him becoming ill in the future. Rick doesn't want to place energy into developing a relationship with someone who will not want to be around him or supportive of him, if he should fall ill.

Elisa, on the other hand, feels differently. She is a thirty-one-year-old woman who has had Crohn's disease since she was sixteen. She goes out with someone for a while before she tells the individual about her disease. She believes that the people whom she dates don't need to know until they have demonstrated to her that they really care about her. Elisa waits until the relationship reaches a certain level of intimacy before she discloses information about her disease or her medical history.

Rick and Elisa have different perspectives on when it is appropriate for them to disclose their disease to the people whom they date. Both Rick and Elisa are comfortable with themselves and their disease processes, but they feel more comfortable disclosing their disease at different times in their relationships. There is no single particular time when it is best to tell somebody about your disease. When the time is right for you to talk about your disease, you'll know it because you'll feel comfortable doing so.

Remember, the right time for you to disclose is when it feels right for you. Living with your disease, and your experience in different situations with previous disclosures, may change your perspective on when to disclose over the course of several dating relationships. Perhaps in your first few relationships you'll want to try talking about it right away. In other dating relationships you might wait a little longer to ascertain the right time for you. It may take a while for you to figure out what's the best approach for you, and that's okay. At times, deciding whether you are going to disclose or not may be more difficult than the coversation itself.

Disclosure: How to Tell

Once you've decided that you're going to tell someone about your disease, you're faced with how to do it. All people with Crohn's disease have their own ways of telling people that work best for them. Here are some suggestions for you that might make your explanation easier.

There are a few questions you can ask someone whom you wish to disclose to that will help with your explanation. For instance, you will want to know if the person has ever heard of Crohn's disease. If so, what do they know about it? Use the information that's provided to you either to confirm his/her ideas or to correct any misunderstandings. If the person hasn't heard of Crohn's disease, offer a general overview. Go over the basic facts about the disease, before you start to explain yours specifically.

Regardless of whether the people you talk to have heard of Crohn's disease or not, having a "standard explanation" of your disease will provide you with a verbal template of sorts. A few sentences briefly explaining what Crohn's disease is, and how it affects you, are usually all that is necessary. Most people are not likely to want the intimate details of your disease; nor will you necessarily want (or need) to state how many times a day you actually use the bathroom. People will want to know how you feel, how your disease is being treated, and when you will feel better. Here is a model of what you might say:

Crohn's disease is a disease of the digestive tract that may affect any part of your digestive system from your mouth to your rectum. The cause of Crohn's disease is unknown. There is no cure for Crohn's disease, but it is not fatal. You can live a normal, healthy life with proper medical treatment. Crohn's disease isn't caused by stress, or the types of food you eat, but stress and the types of food eaten can make the symptoms worse. My disease is located _____. It is being treated with _____. I know that my disease is active when _____ (list your symptoms). What else would you like to know?

You may choose to be more specific, depending on whom you are speaking with. Sometimes people will ask if you are in pain, or what it feels like to have the disease. You may choose to say something like this:

Have you ever had a twenty-four-hour virus, or a flu with diarrhea? Sometimes you may feel lethargic, weak, achy, and physically tired. Active Crohn's disease is like having a twenty-four-hour flu every day. Some days are better than others. But that's sort of what it feels like.

When people ask you if it goes away, as often happens when you tell people that you have an illness, you might decide to say the following:

Crohn's disease is a chronic illness, which means that it will be in my body for the rest of my life. But that doesn't mean it will be active or that I will be sick for the rest of my life. Crohn's disease has both active and inactive periods. Medication is used to control the disease activity, so that I will be able to feel better. The disease can remain inactive for months and/or years at a time. Everyone's body and disease process is different. If you talk to ten different people with Crohn's disease, you are likely to hear ten different versions of 1) how the disease is manifested in the body; 2) how long the disease was active and/or inactive; and 3) differences in treatment. Where the disease is located affects how it is treated by doctors. My disease is located _____, which is why it is being treated with _____.

These are some of the ways you may choose to tell others about your disease. There aren't any right or wrong ways to tell people. Figuring out what is right for you is what's important to both your physical and emotional health.

Disclosure: When It Is Not Appropriate

Now that you've an idea about who, when, and how you might tell someone about your disease, there are also situations in which it might not be appropriate to tell. You want people to know about your disease when their having the information can be helpful to you, or helpful to the people around you by virtue of their interaction with you. You don't want to tell others when it is not relevant, or in situations where you're not comfortable.

There are some situations where it is simply unnecessary to inform others of your disease because it isn't relevant to the activity and/or the situation in which you are involved. For example, just because you and a friend do your food shopping together doesn't mean you have to tell your friend that you have Crohn's disease. When you are at a wedding or other formal affair, you certainly don't need to talk about your disease at the dinner table in order to control what you put into your mouth. This is not to say that you can't talk about your disease, simply that it might not be appropriate to do so.

You may not want to discuss your disease in situations where you are not comfortable. If you are uncomfortable in a given situation that has nothing to do with your disease process, your presentation of your disease in that context might become biased to reflect your lack of comfort with the situation as opposed to your disease.

Hopefully, you want people to feel comfortable with you. If you demonstrate your comfort with your disease by talking about it in a matter-of-fact way, you are more likely to get reactions that reflect your presentation. Some people may be able to view your disease through your eyes, and perhaps you may be able to see your disease differently, through their eyes, as it were.

Chapter 8

Crohn's Disease: What It Means to Others

So, maybe you've told people about your disease, maybe not. What's important to try to remember is that you have control over what information people have about you. Other people will react to you in ways that you've demonstrated as important to you. This chapter focuses on the feelings that you may have when talking about your disease with the people who are important in your life, as well as their possible reactions to you. It also discusses partner relationships, sexuality, and gynecological issues as they pertain to your disease activity.

Reactions of Others

You and the people you decide to tell about your disease process have reactions to discussing your illness and your feelings surrounding it. How you present your illness to others has a great deal to do with how people will respond to you. For instance, if you are emotional or upset when discussing your disease (as is only natural at times), the people with whom you're speaking may become upset for you. Think about how you might feel if someone you cared about was talking to you about a situation they found to be distressing. How would you react? The next section of this chapter discusses a few of the possible emotions you and the people in your life might have regarding your disease.

Concern and Worry

You and the people you know may experience concern and worry about your disease. You may feel this way for a number of reasons. First, you may be worried and concerned about your physical health, especially when you aren't feeling well. Second, you may be worried and concerned about the need to tell someone in your life about your disease. Questions may arise in your mind such as: What will they think? How will they react? Will our relationship change? Naturally, these kinds of questions may be a cause of concern for you, which may increase your anxiety level. Third, you may be concerned about the effects the disease may have on your relationships with others, or if there will be any effect at all.

The people in your life may also experience worry and concern. People who love and care about you want you to be happy and healthy. When you're not feeling well, they may become concerned about you. Those who know about your disease may ask you questions about your disease and how you're feeling because they are concerned. Family members, especially, may demonstrate their concerns to you, in both direct and indirect ways. For instance, there may be some members of your family who will say to you "How's your Crohn's?" (direct concern), and others who might ask you "How have you been feeling? You eating okay/sleeping all right?" (indirect concern).

Regardless of how the concern manifests, these types of feelings are not uncommon for family members. These feelings are likely similar to feelings that *you* may have had as a child when a parent or sibling was ill. Think about how you might feel in such a situation today, for a limited period of time, such as when your child has a cold. Now think about how the people around you might feel worrying about you *all* of the time. Talking about your own concerns as they relate to your relationships will give the people in your life the opportunity to express their concerns as well. Mutual exploration of feelings about the disease and its influence (or lack thereof) on your relationships will help you incorporate your disease into your life.

Discussion Helps

One effective way to handle these types of concerns is to discuss them honestly and openly with the people who are involved. Neither you nor the people in your life are mind readers. You cannot predict how people will react to you, nor can others be expected to know what your concerns are, unless you express them. Open discussion of how you're feeling, what your concerns are, and how the people in your life can be of help to you may alleviate the worry and anxiety you experience about the effect of your disease on your relationships.

For example, Harry is a forty-two-year-old man who was recently diagnosed with Crohn's disease. His wife went with him to the doctor when the disease was explained to him. But Harry has difficulty communicating his concerns and feelings about the disease, in part because not enough time has passed for him to appreciate the potential impact of the disease. His wife, Margaret, on the contrary, is constantly asking him how he feels and what he has eaten.

Recently, Harry and his wife, Margaret, sat down and discussed how she could be of assistance to him. One of Harry's concerns was that he was physically tired all the time, preventing the two of them from engaging in sexual activity as they had all through their married life together. He was worried about his wife's physical needs. She was concerned about his eating and she was worried about his physical health. She, however, wasn't at all concerned about their sexual activity, as she was completely focused on helping him to feel better. Harry wasn't concerned about his eating, because he knew that he was doing the best he could, and he didn't want his wife constantly asking him about his eating habits, which bothered him. Harry told Margaret not to worry so much about his eating habits. He said that it wasn't helpful to him to have her ask him questions all the time. Margaret told him not to worry about their sex life, as that was not a concern of hers. By discussing their feelings, both Harry and his wife were able to alleviate their concerns about each other.

Helplessness and Frustration

Other feelings that you and the people in you life may experience include helplessness and frustration. You may feel helpless about your disease, because sometimes when you're sick, it feels as though there isn't anything you can do to help yourself. No matter what you eat, or what medication you take, it may not ease your symptoms as much as you'd like. When you are sick for long periods of time, you may feel as though your disease activity has control over you, instead of the other way around.

When you feel as though the disease has taken over your life, it can be very frustrating. You don't want to be sick. You don't want to feel physically ill. You take your medication. You eat the foods that you can digest, and you still may not feel that much better. Sometimes Crohn's disease can remain active for weeks and months at a time, which can lead to increased feelings of frustration and helplessness (not to mention, depression, anxiety, and so forth). Also, feelings of frustration and helplessness, in turn, may lead to increased fear and/or anger. Did you ever get angry with someone, and then realize that your anger was really about your disease and not about the person? That is not unusual, everyone displaces anger from time to time. When you're feeling physically ill, however, your tolerance and patience may not be what they usually are and, consequently, you may become even more frustrated with yourself and your disease.

The people in your life may also experience helplessness and frustration. When you watch someone you love and/or care for feeling ill or you see them in physical pain, and know that there is nothing that you can do to help alleviate it, that may bring up even more intense feelings of helplessness and frustration. Try to imagine what it would be like for you if the situation were reversed. What would you feel? What do you think would be helpful to you in that situation? Can you implement the helping thoughts you might be having and be of assistance to yourself and the people around you? Remember, how you handle the helplessness and frustrations that may arise as a consequence of your disease is, in the end, up to you. You have control over how you cope with your feelings, other people, and all the different situations that might arise.

Handling Helplessness

There are no simple solutions for fighting the helplessness that people experience when they have any chronic illness, including Crohn's disease. You choose to deal or cope with your disease in a way that's unique to you and your disease process. Do you remember the Serenity Prayer from chapter 6? When you're feeling frustrated because of your disease, those three sentences may be helpful to you, as well as remembering that your disease won't be active *forever*. It *will* quiet down in time. So, try to remain hopeful and positive.

Sometimes, taking life one day at a time can aid you by keeping you from submerging yourself in worry about the future of your disease. Dealing just with the events of each day as it happens prevents you from becoming overwhelmed with the possibility of overthinking the situation. You do have control over how you cope with your disease. Coping one day at a time, especially during those times when you are feeling badly, will assist you in managing both your symptoms and your life.

Care and Consideration

Michelle and her husband, Lee, scheduled a two-week vacation for themselves in Europe. The trip was planned about three months ahead of time. Michelle has had Crohn's disease for most of their married life (five out of the seven years they have been married). They were really looking forward to the vacation, but exactly one month before they were to leave for Europe, Michelle's disease became active. She became very concerned that she wouldn't feel well enough to travel. After all the planning that she had done for the two of them, she couldn't believe her disease was acting up.

Michelle was going to the bathroom frequently (eight times a day) and occasionally waking up in the middle of the night in pain. She didn't know what to do. Lee was also concerned, but he felt that they should wait and see. As time went on, Michelle's symptoms worsened; she was unable to digest even the most basic of foods. She was afraid to fly or to eat foreign food, and she didn't want to go if she wouldn't be able to leave the hotel. Lee was both supportive and encouraging; he didn't want them to go on vacation if Michelle couldn't enjoy herself. As their travel date approached, Michelle still was feeling only somewhat better, despite medications that she had recently started taking.

Michelle tried to take her disease activity one day at a time. Each day, she told herself that she would feel better. Although this helped her on a daily basis, she still didn't think she would be able to vacation in Europe with Lee as they had planned. After some discussion, they both decided to postpone the trip until such time that Michelle could travel and enjoy herself. Both were disappointed, but they knew that they'd eventually get to go. Michelle felt both frustrated and help-less; their wonderfully planned vacation had been delayed.

Sometimes the disease activity in your body will influence your life in ways that you wish it wouldn't. That's part of the frustration and helplessness that living with a chronic illness brings with it. Try to remember that it's not only you who's feeling the frustration and the helplessness. You're not alone. The people in your life may feel it as well, and talking about it with each other may be quite helpful.

Taking each day as it comes helps you to focus on the moment, not the lifetime. Lee and Michelle did this as best they could, deciding to postpone their trip until they could maximize their enjoyment. Sure, Michelle's disease activity affected their plans. However, postponing their vacation was also another opportunity for the couple to demon-strate the love, compassion, faith, and trust that they have for one another.

Effects on Relationships

There are both direct effects (e.g., fatigue, constant diarrhea, abdomi-nal pain) and indirect effects (e.g., side effects of medication, conse-quences of surgery) of Crohn's disease that may disrupt your interpersonal relationships and your sexual functioning. The direct effects of your disease like constant fatigue, chronic diarrhea and/or abdominal pain, as previously discussed, might affect your mood and your behaviors. You may not feel sociable or sexual. Indirect effects of some of the medications you take also may contribute to your lack of sociability or sexual desire. For instance, some medications can cause oral infections like candidiasis, or thrush (Gerson and Triadafilopoulos 2000). You may feel aversion to even the simple act of kissing, as a consequence of such a side effect.

Discussing your relationship and your sexuality in the context of your disease activity will open communication between you and your partner, and will facilitate your adjustment to living with your disease. Maybe you don't discuss such issues (i.e., your sexuality, your feel-ings about your body, and the effect of your disease on your relation-ships) much. Perhaps you do. The more you can discuss the various effects the disease may be having on your relationships with others, the less likely the disease is to become an impediment to those relationships.

Marriage and Partnerships

When you are in a committed relationship, whether it is a formal marriage or a committed partnership, you've likely developed certain expectations inherent in the "committed" component of your relationship. Both you and your partner have chosen to implement the expectation of commitment for "better or worse," so to speak. Consideration of your disease and both of your feelings about it may help to minimizing the influence of the disease on your relationship. That is, if you openly discuss your thoughts, your feelings, and your concerns about the possible and/or potential effects of the disease on your relationship, you may be more able to comfort and support one another during trying times, thus minimizing the effects of the disease.

When you can discuss so many intimate details about your lives with each other, your disease may not have that large an influence on your relationship at all. However, when your information about your disease and your feelings about it are unknown, that may lead to difficulties that might not otherwise arise. For instance, perhaps you haven't told your partner that when you experience an increase in your symptoms, you become irritable. Then, your partner is more likely to take your increased irritability personally, when it is actually caused by your increased disease symptoms. Talking about your symptoms and your feelings about your disease with your partner may prevent unnecessary miscommunications from occurring.

Impact on Relationships

Matt and Marion are a couple in their late twenties who have been married for four years. Marion has active Crohn's disease. Matt requested couple's therapy because of his wife's "withdrawal" during her periods of disease activity. Marion has had Crohn's disease for approximately twelve years, and she has been controlling the disease activity successfully with medication therapy since her diagnosis. Recently, she experienced a flare-up involving frequent diarrhea, abdominal pain, and urgency causing her to have occasional "accidents." Matt reported that she has become increasingly withdrawn, lethargic, and moody subsequent to her disease becoming active. They have not had intercourse since her flare-up, which was two months ago.

Marion had difficulties discussing her relationship and her feelings about their sexual life. Matt reported that when Marion is sick, she avoids physical affection and is unwilling to discuss her feelings pertaining to her distinct change in behavior. Marion stated that her behavior changes were due to feeling tired and lethargic as a result of her frequent defecation. Matt said that he was frustrated and hurt by Marion's behavior, and that he felt rejected. He described their relationship this way: "It's different when she doesn't feel well. She doesn't let me in and I don't know what to do about it. I don't know what to do to make her feel better."

Matt experiences difficulty with Marion's avoidance because he feels helpless, and wants to relieve her sick feelings. He feels that Marion isolates herself as if "her problem" is not "their problem." Although Matt understands her lack of sexual desire and he demonstrates compassion for her, he feels shut out. He also noted that when she feels well, she acts as though the disease does not exist and doesn't discuss it at those times either.

Marion does feel as though she is a "different person" when her disease is active. She isolates herself due to her lack of sexual desire and her inability to identify and communicate her feelings to Matt. Moreover, Matt reported that if Marion would simply state how she felt, he would feel as though he were a part of "her world."

Matt and Marion illustrate the communication difficulties that can arise between partners due to a lack of communication about both the disease activity and the feelings surrounding it. Their story demonstrates both the direct effects of the disease (frequent diarrhea and abdominal pain) and the indirect effects (lethargy and fatigue) that disease activity can have on both relationships and sexuality.

Singles and Dating

Due to the fact that many people who have Crohn's disease are diagnosed in their late teens and early twenties, there are many young, single people with Crohn's. Consequently, singles with Crohn's, who are dating, are likely to encounter different types of emotional challenges than those in committed relationships. In partnerships like marriage, a certain level of trust and intimacy has already been established, to say nothing of the love and compassion that already exist between a couple, prior to a diagnosis.

When you are single and dating, trust and emotional intimacy have to be first created and then maintained. If you have Crohn's, forming new relationships may be difficult because you might fear rejection. "Hidden" behaviors, such as chronic diarrhea and abdominal pain, may be especially difficult for you to discuss because it is unclear when you might feel safe enough to disclose such information. You may want to establish some level of trust and closeness before contemplating disclosure (Basson 1998).

The length of time you date someone before revealing that you have Crohn's disease is up to you. Often the timing of your disclosure will depend on how active your disease is, how much you enjoy spending time with the person, and what your own comfort level is with your disease. You may choose to speak about your disease on your first or second date, or you may choose to wait until the relationship becomes more serious (as discussed in chapter 7).

Only you can know when you are most comfortable talking about your disease and your experiences surrounding it. However, *not telling* someone you are dating also can become a source of anxiety. Anticipating having that kind of conversation with someone you are dating may make you nervous. If that is the case, try to remember that you can't control other people's reactions to you or to your disease.

What you can do is control your presentation of your disease to the person you are dating by being comfortable with it. Furthermore, consider seriously whether you want to date someone who might not be able to handle the possibility that you may become sick one day. As was previously discussed, people will take their lead from you. If you don't think it is big deal, the person you're telling is not likely to think it is such a big deal either.

Sexuality

Sexuality is almost as private an activity as defecation is. Sex is a topic that piques people's interest, however, private though it may be. As a topic of discussion, defecation doesn't hold the same allure. Unfortunately, Crohn's disease may have an impact on your sexual feelings, due to a lack of desire as a consequence of disease activity, or to a lack of energy as a consequence of disease activity. Perhaps your disease doesn't affect your desire for sex at all, especially in the context of dating, but it may affect your feelings about yourself.

Sometimes the insecurity about having an "accident" or leakage during the act of sexual intercourse can strongly inhibit your sexual motivation (Basson 1998).

Deborah's Dilemma

Deborah, a thirty-six-year-old woman, has been dating Eric for about a month. She has had Crohn's disease for the past two years and, although she uses the bathroom several times a day, her disease has been controlled with medication. Deborah and Eric have been on several dates. During the time the two have spent together, there hasn't been an opportunity for Deborah to mention the disease in the context of their conversation.

Deborah reported that she uses religion as an example. She doesn't tell the people whom she dates about her religious background unless it comes up in conversation, and she takes the same approach with her disease. However, the more time she spends with Eric, and the more she enjoys his company, the greater her fear about telling him about her Crohn's becomes. Deborah is afraid that he won't want to date her anymore. She also thinks that if Eric stops dating her for that reason, then she doesn't want to get involved with him in a long-term relationship. Although Deborah wants to spend more time with Eric and get to know him better, the longer she waits to tell him, the more difficult it becomes for her.

Deborah's conflicted feelings about whether or not to tell Eric about her disease exemplify the potential difficulties that may arise with single people. It's not always easy to become vulnerable with someone whom you don't know very well. Thus, being comfortable with who you are and how your disease affects you assists in decreasing difficulties such as those noted above. Deborah finally did tell Eric about her disease. Afterwards, she said, "If I hadn't said anything to him about my illness, I would still be feeling very nervous. I am glad I told him when I did; now I don't have to worry about it anymore."

Women's Issues

There are some topics regarding Crohn's disease that apply specifically to women. Concerns about gynecological issues and pregnancy are two such topics. As you continue reading, remember that these topics may *not* apply to you and your disease. The information in this next section discusses possibilities—not probabilities.

Gynecology

The two main areas that affect women in particular are concerns about gynecological issues and pregnancy. As a rule, ulcerative colitis does not affect the gynecological regions of the body; however, approximately 25 percent of all Crohn's disease patients incur some sort of gynecological difficulty (James 1993). For these women, the difficulties that might be experienced are both physically painful and emotionally troublesome.

The gynecological complications of Crohn's disease include irregularities in the menstrual cycle, as well as long delays, and amenorrhea, pelvic masses, or occasionally tubo-ovarian abscesses (James 1993). Treatments for these complications usually begin with medications such as antibiotics and immunosuppressives. These complications may cause both pain and discomfort during intercourse (James 1993). Additionally, abscesses and fistulas in the rectal area may interfere with a woman's ability to engage in intercourse and/or sexual activities.

Pregnancy and Inflammatory Bowel Disease (IBD)

Due to the fact that the peak age ranges of IBD and pregnancy coincide, it is likely that there will be an increasing number of pregnant women with IBD (Adler 1992; Korelitz 1998). Some women may become concerned about the impact of Crohn's disease on fertility, pregnancy, and the risk of inheritance (Adler 1992; Saubermann and Wolf 1999; Kane 1999). Generally, fertility is unaffected (Saubermann and Wolf 1999; Kane 1999; Burakoff 1993). At least 80 percent of women will have normal reproductive function and give birth to normal, healthy full term infants (Saubermann and Wolf 1999; Burakoff 1993; Botoman, Bonner, and Botoman, 1998; Burakoff 1995). (In men, sulfasalazine may cause reversible changes in sperm that may lead to a temporary decrease in fertility; however, the new 5-ASA compounds do not appear to affect sperm or fertility (Saubermann and Wolf 1999).)

According to Burakoff (1995), disease activity, not drug therapy, accounts for the majority of complications during pregnancy. In addition, for those women who undergo multiple operations for Crohn's disease, scar tissue surrounding the fallopian tubes and the ovaries may result in immobility of fallopian tubes, and lead to infertility. In these instances, in vitro fertilization may be necessary.

Active disease is not a contraindication to pregnancy, as it can be controlled with medication therapy. There is, however, two to three times greater likelihood of spontaneous abortion or pre-term birth in women with active disease (Saubermann and Wolf 1999; Burakoff 1993, 1995). Consequently, some physicians recommend that pregnancy be delayed until the disease activity becomes quiescent (Baird, Narendranathan, and Sandler 1990). The risk to the fetus is greater due to the activity of your disease, not to the medications used in your treatment. Moser, Okun, Mayes, and Bailey (2000) found that active inflammation in pregnant women is a significant predictor of small gestational age of neonates. (That is, if your disease is active when you are pregnant, there is a possibility that your newborn will be small for its developmental age.) Hence, when you are pregnant, you might consider the effects of your disease on your pregnancy, the effects of your pregnancy on your disease, and potential risks to your unborn child. Certainly, proper nutrition and medical monitoring will also be of assistance to you when you are pregnant.

In Crohn's disease, the relapse rate for inactive disease in pregnant women is approximately 27 percent (Saubermann and Wolf 1999). Relapses of disease activity usually occur in the first trimester or following delivery in Crohn's disease patients. Approximately 33 percent of women with Crohn's will notice an exacerbation of symptoms (Saubermann and Wolf 1999). The risk of flare-up of the disease in future pregnancies is unknown.

Some women may want to avoid using any medications during their pregnancy; however, it may become necessary to take medications in order to maintain your health. Maintaining remission is very important during the course of a pregnancy (Burakoff 1995). Most of the medications used are safe during pregnancy and breast-feeding (Saubermann and Wolf 1999). However, those of you with perianal or anal disease, might consider a cesarean section, rather than a vaginal delivery, with the hope of avoiding rectal complications.

Pregnancy and Crohn's

Joan is a married thirty-seven-year-old woman who was diagnosed with Crohn's disease at the age of twenty-three. Over the course of the last fourteen years, her disease activity has waxed and waned but it was controlled with medication therapy. When Joan and her husband decided they wanted a child, Joan's disease was quiescent, but controlled with a maintenance dosage of a 5-ASA compound. Joan stopped taking her medication on her own, as she did not want to be on medication if pregnancy occurred. Shortly thereafter Joan became pregnant.

In the middle of her first trimester, she began having symptoms that included painful diarrhea and abdominal pain. Her physician placed her back on a 5-ASA compound and monitored her nutrition closely to maintain Joan's nutritional intake and that of her fetus. Due to lethargy, Joan spent a substantial amount of time in bed during the last two months of her pregnancy. Although the baby was born a healthy, full-term infant, Joan's symptoms increased after she delivered, as did her need for medication.

Joan's situation illustrates that, with proper medical management, a healthy full-term infant can be delivered to a woman with Crohn's with only minor difficulties. However, Joan's case also exemplifies the difficulties that you may encounter as a result of not wanting to harm your unborn child. In her desire not to harm her unborn child with medication, she placed her own health at risk. Discussion and consultation with your physician is always helpful in these situations.

Sexual Functioning in Surgical Patients

For those of you who undergo surgical interventions for your disease, social and sexual functioning may also become a concern. An estimated 70 percent of Crohn's disease patients will require surgery (Sachar 1997). Several studies looked at social and sexual functioning in women postoperatively (Bambrick, Fazio, and Hull 1996; Damgaard, Wettergren, and Kirkegaard 1995; Metcalf, Dozios, and Kelly 1986; Seidel, Peach, Newman, and Sharp 1999; Tianen, Matikainen, and Hiltunen 1999; Scaglia, Bronsino, Canino, et al. 1993; Scaglia, Delaini, and Hulten 1992). Most of the investigations reported that due to improved general health postoperatively, women experienced enhanced sexual functioning (Bambrick, Fazio, Hull, and Puce 1996; McLeod 1997; Metcalf, Dozios, and Kelly 1986).

In the study conducted by Damgaard, Wettergren, and Kirkegaard (1995) it was found that sexual functioning improved after surgery. In their study, 35 percent of women (N=23) reported that their frequency of intercourse increased, none reported a decrease in sexual functioning, and 16 percent reported an increased quality of orgasm. In people who have ostomies, poor rapport between partners following surgery correlated with poor sexual relations prior to surgery (Huish, Kumar, and Stones 1989), thus indicating the importance of effective communication and support in interpersonal relationships. Gloeckner (1983) reported that patients wished their partners had been included in sexual counseling postoperatively.

Consequences of Surgery

Nancy is a thirty-four-year-old married woman with Crohn's disease. She was initially diagnosed with ulcerative colitis, and underwent an ileoanal anastamoses at the age of thirteen. Some years later, doctors recognized that she had Crohn's disease due to her symptoms of recurring diarrhea, abdominal pain, and extra-intestinal manifestations. Multiple resections over the years resulted in an extensive amount of scar tissue attaching to one of her Fallopian tubes.

Three years ago, an ileostomy replaced her J-pouch, and within six months, her symptoms returned again. A fallopian tube required removal. She and her husband would like to have a child and, although her fallopian tube was removed, Nancy will be able to carry a baby full-term with in vitro fertilization. She decided she needed some psychotherapy due to her frustration with her disease.

Nancy had been married twice prior to her current marriage. Although she has had Crohn's since her childhood, she reported that she always has had difficulty discussing her disease with her marital/relationship partners. Moreover, she stated that, in all of her marriages, the topic of her illness was rarely discussed.

She underwent surgery for her ileostomy a short while after her third marriage, and stated only that it had been "difficult," but even during the therapy sessions, she was uncomfortable communicating her feelings. In therapy, Nancy reported many concerns regarding her perception of her sexuality. Some sessions later, she said that she had

had an affair with another man simply to see whether she would be sexually desirable to someone other than her husband "despite the ostomy."

Although she reported that sexual intercourse was "good" with her husband, she stated that she feels as though "the bag" has changed her sexual repertoire. For example, she said that certain positions, which used to be enjoyable, are no longer comfortable for her. She also stated that she does not communicate her sexual wants and needs to her partner for fear that it will not be well received. She said that when she feels well, she does not like to discuss her disease with her husband. "When it isn't bothering me, I like to forget it exists."

Although Nancy was pleased to learn that she may still become pregnant, her anxiety and depression focus on potential problems that might occur during her pregnancy. When you have an illness that's associated with social stigma, difficulties incorporating the disease into your life may arise. Nancy separates herself from her illness and, when she feels healthy, she functions as if the disease does not exist. Unfortunately, her difficulties communicating her feelings to her partner thwart her acceptance of the reality of her disease. If Nancy discussed her feelings about her sexuality with her husband, she might not have felt the need to seek affirmation of her sexuality outside of her marriage. Moreover, her decision to withhold her feelings does not help her to accept her disease either by herself or with her partner as a part of their life together.

Crohn's disease as it relates to interpersonal relationships, sexuality, pregnancy, and surgery are subjects that you might want to explore and discuss with your physicians and significant others to facilitate your own adjustment to the illness (Gerson and Triadafilopoulos 2000). Effective communication between you and your partner(s), and between you and your physician will be of great assistance to you when dealing with the topics discussed throughout this chapter.

Moreover, your sexual partners can play key roles in helping you adjust to your illness if you allow it. Whenever possible, you might include your partner(s) in addressing the relationship and sexual issues that might arise as a consequence of your disease activity. By addressing the problems and fears pertaining to your relationship and your sexuality, future potential difficulties may become a nonissue. Support from the people in your life does help. The next chapter discusses social support, and explains why it can be of benefit to you.

Chapter 9

Social Support

"Social support" is the term frequently used to describe additional resources that people may access to assist in adjusting to living with disease, illness, and/or other difficulties. In fact, social support is of great help to those people living with *any* type of medical or psychological difficulty, regardless of the disease or illness (e.g. cancer, depression, HIV, or bereavement).

The social support networks that individuals can access are often crucial to the adjustment process. Although it is important for you to help yourself, it is also valuable to receive assistance from others. Given that Crohn's disease can be difficult to discuss, even, at times, with your own physician, the people with whom you choose to share your experiences may influence how you handle your disease.

Crohn's disease may, for the most part, not be easy to discuss. Why? Some of the reasons have already been discussed. The bottom line is that no one wants to talk about shitting: it is that simple. Yet, everyone, no matter who they are, where they come from, what language they speak, and/or whether or not they have the disease, shits. Unfortunately, for those with Crohn's disease, you have to talk about it and deal with it, as much as you might not want to. After all, who actually wants to talk about a disease that causes you to go to the bathroom all the time? You are *doing* it enough, why should you have to talk about it, too?

About Social Support

There are five definitions of the word "support" in *Webster's Collegiate Dictionary*. The first four focus on the ability to "bear and maintain," while the fifth emphasizes the ability to provide aid and assistance. You may think of support only in terms of verbal communication. People talking with one another may be the most natural type of social support. Support group meetings are filled with small groups of people talking with one another. Discussing your experiences with other people *is* a form of social support. When you talk about your disease on the phone with your friend, and s/he listens to you, that's social support. When you attend a support group meeting, that, too, is considered social support.

Nonverbal communication, such as body language, warmth, empathy, and others' facial expressions, also appears to have an impact on your sense of feeling supported. Not surprisingly, actions speak louder than words. For instance, think about the daily interactions you have with others and how you communicate with them. People communicate just as much, if not more, through nonverbal communication or body language as they do through verbal language. (See chapters 6 and 7 for a discussion of nonverbal communication.) You need to be aware of your nonverbal communications when you are trying to access social support, whether you obtain it from family and friends, or from members of your community. The effectiveness of your communications both verbally and nonverbally, may be instrumental in obtaining and accessing social support.

Why Social Support Is Important

Feeling as though you are supported (i.e., having a group of people to depend on), helps you adjust to living with the disease. It assists you in feeling understood, and it reinforces the fact that you are not alone. Having others to support you is also helpful to your own self-acceptance. There is nothing "wrong with you" or who you are, simply because you have a medical illness. Although having an illness like Crohn's may encourage feelings of "being different," talking to others will help you to realize that many people share your experiences, even if in different contexts. When other people demonstrate their understanding of you and your disease, that can and does tend to make those with Crohn's disease feel better.

When other people understand and accept you as you are, that helps you to adjust to and accept your disease *as a part of* who you are. Happily, there are those who will likely consider and provide appropriate support to you, people who will help you out when you cry out for "aid and assistance," and they will rally around you to help you find a way to "bear and maintain."

It is valuable and healthy to talk about your disease experiences with others. You can gain support from those who listen to you, and obtain information by listening to others. Mutual sharing of experiences is a cooperative effort. Many people find that sharing their experiences with others who have the disease is easier than talking to those without the disease because "people who don't have the disease don't understand." People without the disease may not have experiences with Crohn's disease, but, certainly, everyone has the capacity to comprehend physical pain and suffering. Try not to discount anyone simply because s/he doesn't have the illness you do.

As mentioned in chapter 7, it is a different experience talking to those with the disease and those without it. If you can effectively communicate your needs and wants, those without the disease can be equally supportive as those with it, just in differing ways. If you are in need of social support for whatever reason, never discount the people around you, especially those who care about you, simply because they don't have the disease.

You may find that there are people who will understand you, and they will validate all the feelings and thoughts you have had regarding your illness. Although it is essential for you to help yourself, there may be times when you simply cannot do it all alone. There may be times when you need other people's assistance, either for physical or emotional reasons. Thus, it is important for you to know what resources are available to you, and how to identify those times when you need to access them. The rest of this chapter will cover these topics: when to access your support system, who constitutes support, and where you can receive support.

When Should You Access Support?

At times, you may require and request support from other people for both physical and emotional reasons. There will be some occasions in which you will need and/or require more support than others. There may be times when you are physically ill, when you experience symptoms of lethargy, fever, and pain that will require you to have physical help getting around places. For example, after an operation, you may need physical help moving around. Physical help isn't the type of assistance that most people like having to ask for or want to receive. Often, when adults feel physically weak, their emotions are fragile, as well. In this context, "fragile" means that the slightest upset may cause a range of emotional reactions from anger to tears to laughter. Think about the times you've had a cold or flu. Were you not both physically and emotionally compromised to some degree?

Asking for help is easier for some people than for others. However, whenever you are physically compromised, it is appropriate to seek support and assistance. Recognizing that you need help and asking for it will be of more use to you over the long haul than "doing it yourself" and suffering the consequences of your actions.

You need support not only when you are physically vulnerable but when you are emotionally vulnerable as well. There may be times when you feel isolated or lonely simply because you think you are the only person in the room with a difficulty or problem like yours. Although isolation may work for some people, the sense of being alone is often accompanied by a feeling of vulnerability. At those times when you feel vulnerable, it is good to seek social support. When will this be? Although you may be more at risk for isolation when you are feeling ill, only you really know when you are feeling vulnerable, alone, and in need of support.

If you experience feelings of isolation and loneliness specifically in regard to your disease, that means it is time for you to start talking to and with other people. It may seem easier to hide from the disease and the disease process. If you don't talk about it, no one has to know that "it" exists. That actually might work for a while, but it won't change the fact that you have the disease. The faster you accept your disease, the greater your ability will be to communicate your thoughts and feelings about it to those around you.

Sources of Support: Who Can Help?

How is support given to you? Whom do you go to for support? There are many different types of people from whom you can derive support when necessary. Sources of support may include, but are not limited to, family, friends, coworkers, and other people with the disease. It is up to you to decide whom you want to include in your support system. However, those people who care about you and who are a part of your life might be among the first people you choose to include. People who care about you, typically, want to help you out in ways that are useful for you. It is up to you, however, to tell them how they can be of assistance.

Although the physician's role is not traditionally thought of as "supporter," some of your greatest supporters are the physicians who monitor and support you through the treatment of your disease. As discussed in chapter 2, effective communication between you and your doctor is necessary for a cooperative relationship to develop. Consequently, "medical support" for those with Crohn's disease requires a collaborative effort between you and your doctor in alliance with the treatment against the disease. Because Crohn's disease is chronic and incurable, the need to develop a long-term supportive relationship between you and your doctors is clearly indicated. Moreover, the chronicity and symptomatology of your disease warrant the establishment of a supportive relationship between you and your doctor.

Anyone who makes you feel better may be classified as a supporter. A friend, family member, coworker, or whoever it is who makes you feel comforted, safe, secure, and provides you with a sense of connection, is support. You know who makes you laugh, puts a smile on your face, and changes your perception of the world (even if only momentarily).

How to Get Social Support

Finding social support is only as difficult as you make it. If you know how to help yourself, you know how to tell others what your needs are. Identify all the people you are going to include in your support system, whether they are family members, friends, or anyone else you know who you think might be of assistance to you. Then, identify those who would be most willing or most likely to help you out in various situations. For instance, there may be certain people whom you feel would be more helpful to you in certain situations than others.

For example, Kevin, a thirty-seven-year-old man has had Crohn's disease for fourteen years. There are times when his disease is more active than others. When his disease is active and he does not feel well, he attends monthly support group meetings, held at a local hospital. When he does feel well, he does not attend the meetings.

He attends the support group meetings when he feels ill for several reasons. First, it is helpful to him to hear about the experiences of others, and how other people handle difficulties similar to his own (e.g., how to handle frequent bathroom use in the workplace). Second, attending support groups makes him feel better because sometimes he has the opportunity to assist other people, too. Finally, Kevin is reminded at the meetings that there are people who live with Crohn's disease in a healthy, well-functioning manner.

Figure out what makes you feel comforted and communicate that to the people in your support system. For example, you could say, "When you do X, I like it because it helps me with Y. Douglas, a twenty-four-year-old man with the disease, used a variation of that "formula" when talking to his girlfriend. He said that when he goes to the bathroom frequently, and he is tired and lethargic, he does not like to be affectionate. He also said that he finds it both comforting and helpful when she rubs his lower back. Consequently, Douglas and his girlfriend have negotiated a way to make Douglas feel supported and understood by his girlfriend, as well as help him to feel better physically and emotionally.

Think of specific ways in which your support system might be of assistance to you and communicate those needs. Try to think of ways to say to your supporter(s) "I like when you do X, because it helps me with Y." For example, if you have a partner who leaves the toilet seat up, you might want to ask him to remember to put it down. You also want to explain to people *why* what they do for you is helpful. In the last example, for instance, you might tell your partner that it is helpful to you to have the toilet seat down, so that when you wake up in the middle of the night to use the toilet, you don't have to sit on the cold porcelain with your bare bottom while you're half asleep.

Explaining to people why certain behaviors are helpful to you will make it easier for them to actually do what you've asked. In a work-related example, if you think that your desk at work is too far from a bathroom, you could explain to your boss that the uncertainty and the sense of urgency you sometimes experience cause you anxiety during the course of the day. Having your desk nearer to a rest room would alleviate the stress of worrying what might happen if the "urge hits" you suddenly.

The Crohn's and Colitis Foundation of America (CCFA)

The Crohn's and Colitis Foundation of America (CCFA) is an organization that originated from a desire to aid and assist those who have Crohn's disease and ulcerative colitis. Its mission is to prevent and cure these diseases through research, and to improve the quality of life of people with these diseases through education and supportive services. The Crohn's and Colitis Foundation of America funds researchers who are interested specifically in these illnesses in an effort to find the cure. The foundation is a nonprofit volunteer health organization, dedicated specifically to these diseases. It runs programs both at the national and local levels to raise money for funding research specifically on Crohn's disease and ulcerative colitis.

There are now over fifty-five chapters and affiliates, many with professional staff at the local level. The organization sponsors many research projects, including studies in Israel and The Netherlands. It also firmly believes in the importance of education. The CCFA publishes books, newsletters, informational pamphlets and, recently, they have developed a scientific journal dedicated specifically to the inflammatory bowel diseases. There are programs throughout the country designed to help raise money for research and education. Walk-a-thons, bowl-a-thons, luncheons, dinners, educational seminars, and training seminars for professionals are some of the many different events that take place throughout the year all over the country.

In addition, CCFA at both the national and local levels has people answering phoned-in, commonly asked questions about Crohn's disease and ulcerative colitis. If you want more information on CCFA, or if you need questions answered, call the national office at 1-800-932-2423. You can also look them up online where you can see for yourself all the services available specifically for people with Crohn's and colitis.

Support Groups

Support groups are frequently used to enable individuals to obtain aid and assistance from one another to address specific problems. The first support group was organized by Joseph Pratt in the early 1900s to decrease depression and increase adherence to medical regimens for people with tubercular disease. In a climate that promotes good health and its maintenance, support groups have become the standard of supplemental care for a plethora of illnesses. Support groups exist for a variety of physical and mental health problems, including drug addictions, smoking cessation, weight control, and bereavement.

Most hospitals provide support groups for people living in the community as well as for those who are in the hospital. Individuals with cardiac problems, cancer, AIDS, inflammatory bowel disease, diabetes, epilepsy, and many other illnesses have access to support groups. There are also psychosocial support groups for single parents, sexual abuse victims, women experiencing menopause, violent offenders, and a variety of other groups. What support entails is often quite complex, given the differing needs and multiple issues presented for consideration in a specific time period.

Occasionally, the *process* of meeting with a group of people with similar problems is a catalyst for change in and of itself. Scientific literature has also demonstrated that the social structure of support groups promotes the expression of relevant emotions, which then acts as a buffer against stress (Antoni and Schneiderman 1998; Antoni, Scneiderman, and Ironson 2000).

When discussing support groups, aid and assistance are identified as the focus of such groups. These types of groups will provide you with helpful information and experiences with other patients with similar problems. Support groups may offer their greatest assistance to you by the mutual cooperation and sharing of information, as well as by giving you a forum to ask questions about other patients' experiences.

Detoxifying your illness in a group setting helps to decrease anxiety and worry, and strengthens your ability to "bear and maintain." Through the support provided to you by the development of your doctor-patient relationship and the support provided to you by a support group, you will have the potential to positively affect both your adjustment to your illness and, ultimately, the course of your disease. Moreover, it is a way to meet others with the disease and to share experiences about the disease process and its treatments.

CCFA Support Groups

The CCFA is the national organization that sponsors local inflammatory bowel disease (IBD) support group meetings through satellite chapters at the local level. Local chapters independently govern their own support group meetings throughout the country. Consequently, support for those with IBD and their families is distributed differently, depending upon the geographic location.

For instance, IBD support groups in some regions of the country meet for two hours per week for twelve consecutive weeks a year. Support groups in other geographic areas hold meetings for two hours monthly each year. Because the duration of time and the structure of support groups are factors that have an impact on the manner in which you receive support, the different methods by which support is allocated require some consideration. Consequently, the CCFA provides a nationwide facilitator training program that provides guidelines to those who lead support groups. Currently, CCFA-sponsored support groups follow these structured guidelines, which allows you to receive the best support possible.

Who runs CCFA support groups? Facilitators for IBD support groups may range from family members and friends of those with IBD, to other patients, or to people who are simply interested in volunteering their time. However, most CCFA support group facilitators are unpaid volunteers who obtain their experience *in situ*, that is, on the site of the support group's meeting place. Facilitators may or may not have IBD disease, and those who do have usually experienced an abundance of medical experiences (hospitalization, surgery, etc.) as a direct result of their disease. Recently, formal training among the facilitators has helped to alleviate any potential errors by both experienced and novice facilitators that may have been made in the past. The CCFA supported a national training workshop of all facilitators nationwide to ensure that support is provided by formally trained individuals. Currently, formal training is required to become a facilitator of a CCFA-sponsored support group.

Why Information About CCFA Is Important

Information about the organization (i.e., what it is and what it does) is important for you so that you have access to an additional knowledgeable resource about your disease. The CCFA can provide accurate, comprehensive information to you, as well as assist you with some of the other topics this book has covered, such as finding a physician's name and/or accessing support in your area. You don't have to be involved with CCFA to know about it and/or to access the organization for information and support (which is why CCFA came to be). Of course, if you want to become involved with the organization, your participation would likely be welcomed.

Getting Involved

The best way to find out about CCFA-sponsored support groups is to call the national office at 800-932-2423 and ask for the number of the local chapter nearest you. You can also ask your doctor if s/he knows of anyone with the disease willing to talk to you. Give your doctor your phone number for the individual to contact you, if s/he chooses. In this way, you don't have to ask your doctor to compromise doctor-patient confidentiality, and you have the benefit of your doctor's referral. Also, you don't place the person you will be speaking to "on the spot" by calling directly.

You might consider calling your local chapter of CCFA at the number provided to you by the national organization. Ask your chapter representative when support group meetings are held, and if they could pass along your phone number to someone who would be willing to speak to you about your disease. If you want to become involved, let the local chapter know that you are willing to become a volunteer; let them know what you will and will not do. As a volunteer, you have the right to choose the activities in which you would like to participate.

Whether you become involved in CCFA or not, whether you attend support groups or not, know that you are not alone. There are many people with Crohn's disease in the world; some of them access social support and some don't. As you've probably figured out by now, what's all right for one individual with Crohn's disease isn't necessarily okay for someone else with the disease. Social support has, nevertheless, been shown to be helpful in reducing depression and feelings of isolation among many medical illnesses, not just Crohn's disease. So, when you are feeling as though you don't want anyone in the world to bother you, try to remember that scientific fact. Also, remember that whatever you decide is right for you, whether it is talking to someone or not, it will be the right decision because you made it.

So, what do you do if you want the world to leave you alone? Well, you allow yourself the time to be alone; temporarily, of course. Always indulge yourself if and when you can, but like anything else in life, do it in moderation. Don't spend three days in your house not answering the phone. Decide what a reasonable time frame would be for you to disengage from the world and, then, when your time is up, re-engage the world. During those times that you feel scared, or insecure, or sad, know that there are other people who have felt as you do, and have gone through difficult times such as the kind you may be experiencing. If you don't want to talk about your disease for the moment, that's okay, but sometimes it might be helpful for you to talk with someone whom you feel is supportive.

Chapter 10

Nutrition and Crohn's Disease: What to Eat

Nutrition, or more specifically, what you "should" eat, is a common topic of discussion for most people with Crohn's disease. Unfortunately, there are no fixed guidelines for the answer to the question "What should I eat?" As you already know, everyone is different, and everyone's disease is different. Some people are lactose-intolerant, some are not. Some people can eat popcorn, some cannot. There are some general guidelines that you can follow, however, that will be helpful in your search for an eating regimen that will work for you. This chapter explains why nutrition is important to you, provides you with suggestions for figuring out a workable eating program, gives you some information on the relationship between your emotions and your eating patterns, and discusses the relationship between your medications and your eating patterns.

Although many physicians commonly suggest special diets for people who have Crohn's disease, one thing is clear: *Food does not cause your disease!* No one food or group of specific foods causes Crohn's disease. Eating certain types of food may cause you to use the bathroom more frequently than you otherwise would, but it doesn't cause your disease. Food exacerbates disease activity or, *if your disease is already active,* it makes it worse. It does not cause you to have the disease, nor does the consumption of any food bring on an active phase of your disease.

Additionally, there is no specific diet that will make your disease go away. You can dine on broiled chicken and chicken broth until the turn of the next century, and it won't make your disease go away (again, my apologies). By now, you must realize that there simply is no "quick fix" for getting rid of your disease. The next section of this chapter will help you to understand why proper nutrition is still important to you, regardless of your disease activity or how frequently you use the toilet. It will also provide you with an idea of how to develop and maintain an eating regimen that works for you as someone living with Crohn's disease.

Why Nutrition Is Important

For starters, nutrition is important to everyone for healthier living. Proper nutrition is especially important for those with Crohn's disease. It is especially important to you because of the type of illness you have in your body, where food can cause you additional difficulties.

When you have adequate and appropriate nutrition, your body receives the correct amounts of nutrients and minerals it needs to function properly. Malnutrition occurs when your body doesn't receive the nutrients and minerals it needs to function properly. When you are malnourished, you may feel lethargic and you may not be able to perform the daily activities your life requires. Malnourished people have a more difficult time resisting infections and fighting infections, and they may experience a lengthier healing process (Greenwood 1992). Specifically, whether or not your disease is active, your body doesn't obtain all the nutrients and minerals that it normally would from ordinary foods if you didn't have this disease.

Malnutrition, Anemia, and Crohn's Disease

Malnutrition is not uncommon; neither is weight loss (Heller 1992). It is easier for you to become dehydrated and nutrient-deficient with Crohn's disease in your body than without it, regardless of whether your disease is active or not. If you are using the bathroom frequently, you may be eating less than you normally do, and the food doesn't stay in your body that long. Or you may be eating more than you usually do, with a feeling of never-ending hunger. Well, your body doesn't absorb the food as it otherwise might (without the disease), barring your unique digestive system. Hence, some people have problems with nutrition regardless of their disease activity, but nutritional problems may arise especially when the disease is active.

For example, a twenty-one-year-old man, Al, appears to be healthy. He has Crohn's disease, and his disease is inactive. He has a healthy appetite and can eat substantial amounts of food at any given meal. He does not experience typical symptoms of active Crohn's disease, such as diarrhea and abdominal cramping. Yet, he is on the slim side. He doesn't use the toilet that frequently, perhaps once or twice a day depending on what he has eaten. However, his physician has told him that he is anemic (meaning that Al lacks a sufficient amount of iron) and wants him to increase his vitamin B12 intake. On the surface, or to the person on the street, it would appear that Al eats well and retains his food. However, he simply isn't obtaining all the nutrients he needs from his diet. Al's anemia might be due to his eating regimen, and not to his illness.

However, because the disease process has an impact on the minerals and nutrients that are absorbed into the body, it is essential for you to maintain a healthy eating regimen, especially when your disease isn't active. When Al monitors his food intake *when he is feeling well*, he is more able to help his immune system if he should become ill *for any reason*, not simply because of his Crohn's disease.

Similarly, by maintaining a healthy diet, you will help yourself in the present *and* in the future should difficulties arise with your disease in the future. As many of you know, when you are constantly going to the bathroom it is difficult to retain the food, much less the nutrients and minerals in the food.

How the Digestive System Works

Digestion is the process by which food, namely nutrients and minerals, are absorbed into the body and broken down into the bloodstream, so that the body can function properly. The digestive system extends from the mouth to the anus, or the rectum. As Crohn's disease can affect any part of your digestive system (i.e., from your mouth to your anus), an understanding of how your digestive system works will be helpful to your understanding of why good nutritional health is integral to your daily lifestyle.

The *mouth* receives the food and reduces it in size via chewing, and mixes it with saliva, which contains digestive enzymes (Greenwood 1992). The *esophagus* is a hollow muscular tube that transports the food from the mouth to the *stomach*. In the stomach, the food is broken down further into liquid form via the addition of enzymes and stomach acids. The liquid produced in the stomach is released into the small intestine at regular intervals, when nutrients and minerals are absorbed and released into the bloodstream.

The *small intestine* is comprised of the duodenum, the jejunum, and the ileum. Each part of the small intestine absorbs the nutrients that have been digested through fingerlike projections called *villi.* (Is ninth-grade biology coming back to you yet?) Once absorbed into the bloodstream as nutrients, they are passed into the bloodstream for delivery to cells throughout the body.

The *pancreas* produces the secretions required for the digestion and absorption of food. The secretions the pancreas makes are released into the duodenum as a reaction to the presence of food. The *liver* produces and secretes bile salts, which aid in the digestion of fats by acting as a detergent. The *gall bladder* stores the bile salts that are not immediately required for digestion.

Material that is not digested travels from your small intestine into your *colon,* or *large intestine*, where water and electrolytes are absorbed, and waste is formed. Waste is matter excreted from the bowel, which consists of unabsorbed food, water, bacteria, and intestinal secretions. At the end of the large intestine is the *rectum*, where waste is stored until it is eliminated by your body.

Because Crohn's disease generally affects portions of the small intestine, poor absorption of nutrients may occur due to the impact of the disease on your body's ability to absorb nutrients efficiently. Thus, decreased nutritional status (malnutrition) may result in your body. This is not to imply that disease in the large intestine is not also associated with malabsorption or malnutrition; it is simply to highlight the reason why eating habits are important to those with Crohn's disease. A poor eating regimen can lead to significant malnutrition, especially when you have active disease.

Nutritional Problems That May Arise

There are four main ways the disease process may influence your digestive system:

- Malabsorption

- Increased secretion and nutrient loss

- Drugs and/or medications affecting nutrients

- Increased need for requirements

Malnutrition may arise from any one or a combination of these processes. It arises more often from poor dietary intake, rather than malabsorption (O'Keefe and Rossner 1994), which is another reason why adhering to a healthy diet is so important to your overall health. Nevertheless, an understanding of the processes by which you may become malnourished will be beneficial to you.

Malabsorption

Malabsorption is the failure of the process by which nutrients are absorbed into the body. It is not uncommon for people with Crohn's disease to become *anemic*, or iron-deficient. When you are anemic, you may have less energy not simply because you are using the bathroom more often, but because you do not have appropriate amounts of iron in your system to provide you with energy. Anemia can be caused by multiple nutritional deficiencies (O'Keefe and Rossner 1994); the most common are iron, B12, and folate. If you are anemic, your doctor might suggest that you take iron supplements to counteract your body's lack of iron.

People with Crohn's disease may become protein-deficient or experience fat malabsorption. The severity of your disease activity may have an influence on your ability to absorb proteins and fats. For example, someone who uses the toilet thirteen times a day is more likely to experience nutritional deficiencies than someone who uses it twice a day. Moreover, fat and proteins may be more difficult for you to digest than pasta or rice, which are carbohydrates.

Calcium is another nutrient that can be lacking among people with Crohn's disease. Typically, people with Crohn's have decreased intake and absorption of calcium, as well as decreased bone mass

(Heller 1992). People may be calcium-deficient for a number reasons. First, those who are lactose-intolerant still require calcium; they just need to get it from sources other than food (i.e., supplements). Second, long-term use of prednisone may result in calcium deficiency, or bone density loss. Third, when you are going to the bathroom frequently for several weeks at a time, your body just doesn't get the nutrition it otherwise would.

Although milk and milk products are often targeted as exacerbating symptoms of Crohn's disease, it is unclear as to whether it is the lactose, the protein, or the fat/fatty acid content that causes the difficulties (Heller 1992). Only you know whether milk and the milk products you consume make you sick or not. How do you know that? By eating those foods, of course. Finding out which foods will agree with your digestive system or not is discussed later in this chapter.

Calcium is of particular concern for women, as the potential to develop osteoporosis can become a cause for concern. Women with Crohn's disease might consider undergoing a bone density test, not because there is anything necessarily wrong, but to ensure that future bone density loss, if it occurs, can be detected. (The physician can compare bone density at a future date to the initial test for evaluative purposes. The initial test establishes a baseline.) This might serve as a precautionary measure for women who are concerned about future bone loss. Most healthy women do not take the recommended daily allowance of calcium (1200 mg a day) (Heller 1992). Thus, calcium supplementation is a good idea. For example, many people take TUMS on a daily basis, a form of calcium carbonate as their calcium supplement.

Sources of Calcium	Sources of Iron
Yogurt	Spinach
Broccoli, green leafy vegetables	Lean cuts of red meat
Tofu	Green leafy vegetables
Canned sardines or salmon	Foods containing vitamin C

Increased Secretion and Nutrient Loss

The disease process in your body may also affect your nutritional status. Your bowel can become inflamed as a result of disease activity. Due to the inflamed motion of the bowel wall, loss of protein occurs. Because of the diarrhea caused by your Crohn's disease, there may be an increased loss of electrolytes and minerals. Loss of blood from the bowel causes increased nutrient loss as well. Some physicians suggest drinking Gatorade because it replenishes the electrolytes in your system.

Increased Need for Nutrients

When you experience nutritional losses, your need for nutrients increases. A cycle develops in which your disease activity increases, your nutritional status decreases, and your need for nutrients increases. For those of you with active disease, symptoms of fever and infection may not be unfamiliar to you. Fevers and/or internal infections also require a larger amount of nutrients than your body normally would need to function. Likewise, your body needs more energy to function because of the infection(s) in your body. Thus, your body's requirements for food increase along with your need for increased amounts of energy just for functioning.

Establishing Nutritional Wellness

Figuring out whether you are nutritionally sound or not is much easier to do than figuring out which foods will upset your stomach. Blood tests can answer specific questions about your nutritional status. If you are concerned about your nutritional status, consult with your doctor about it, and ask for blood work if it will assuage your concerns. Also, blood tests can provide you with a good sense of the type of nutrients and minerals that you require to keep yourself feeling healthy and well. If you are concerned that your daily eating habits are not meeting your body's nutritional needs, seek assistance from a nutritionist who knows about Crohn's disease. Seeking help from a nutritionist who does not know about Crohn's disease can cause you greater difficulties.

Medications Affecting Nutrient Intake

The following list highlights some of the medications that may cause nutritional deficiency. This does *not* mean that if you are taking these medications, you will become nutrient deficient.

- Prednisone reduces calcium absorption and increases the breakdown of protein.

- Sulfasalazine (Azulfidine) decreases folate absorption.

For example, Mara, a thirty-seven-year old woman, has had Crohn's disease for twenty years. She has been on and off prednisone and sulfasalazine for many years. Her disease activity has repeatedly waxed and waned over the twenty-year period of her illness. Although Mara has always been on the thin side, her most recent bout with Crohn's disease left her severely malnourished. So, even though Mara has been feeling better, and her disease activity is under control, she sought the advice of a nutritionist in her community.

Mara wanted to be able to eat in a manner that provided her body with all of the nutrients and minerals it needed to function as best she could. The nutritionist she consulted, however, did not know what Crohn's disease was, or how the illness process worked. Consequently, the nutritionist provided her with quite a well-balanced eating regimen, but it was not one that Mara could tolerate. For instance, salads and vegetables comprised a substantial portion of the eating regimen. Makes sense, right? Salads and vegetables comprise a well-balanced eating protocol.

However, Mara couldn't tolerate foods such as romaine lettuce, broccoli, and cauliflower as they caused her bowel symptoms to increase (e.g., diarrhea). Mara followed the nutritionist's regimen only for a short while, because her body reacted adversely to the foods that had been suggested, and unpleasant physical symptoms arose. Mara's diarrhea increased. She visited her physician, who suggested that she should try a low-residue diet to try to decrease the bowel symptoms. (Low-residue diets will be discussed shortly.) When Mara eliminated the salads and vegetables from her diet, her physical symptoms diminished. She had learned a valuable lesson. When you seek guidance regarding living a healthier lifestyle, the person providing assistance to you must have some knowledge about your disease. The greater the knowledge about the disease, the greater your assurance that you will receive the best care possible.

Total Parenteral Nutrition (TPN)

Total parenteral nutrition is oral nutritional therapy for people who are extremely sick. Although TPN is one way of becoming nutritionally sound, it is not an option you would elect unless you were very ill. This type of treatment is prescribed by your physician and involves feeding yourself through a tube that is inserted into one of your veins. It is quite similar to an intravenous tube, only you receive nutrients instead of medications through it. Sometimes TPN is prescribed to help give your bowel a rest. Sometimes it is prescribed to help your body receive nutrients in addition to the food you are already eating. Total parenteral nutrition is not a type of dietary regimen that you want to follow, it is a nutritional regimen that assists with survival. So what you want to do, ideally, is to eat foods that you can tolerate, foods that you enjoy, that provide your body with the nutrients and minerals it needs to function properly.

Finding the Right Foods

When you are initially diagnosed, you may not know which foods will cause you to have increased diarrhea. Be patient. After a while you will come to know those foods you can and cannot eat. Because everyone is different, much of your knowledge about which foods you can tolerate will come from your experiences living with the disease. You will come to know which foods you can eat endlessly (like broiled chicken) and, perhaps, never get sick from. You will come to know which foods will give you pain and diarrhea (e.g., broccoli). You will also find out which foods will give you pain and diarrhea, *and* that you will eat anyway. Why? You enjoy them too much to give them up forever (e.g., popcorn). As you read the next section, you must understand that the examples provided may or may not apply to you. They relate to foods that *most* people have difficulty digesting, but may be fine for *you* to eat. For instance, in the examples above, broiled chicken may make you sick, and broccoli and popcorn may be tolerated by your digestive tract. Remember, this book provides guidelines and information on what happens to *many* people with Crohn's disease, not to *all* people with Crohn's disease.

Trial and Error Eating

Trial and error eating is just what it says. You try certain foods and if they make you symptomatic or sick, you don't eat them again.

This sounds too simple to be the truth, nevertheless, it is. There are certain foods that you will find make you feel sick consistently when you eat them, and you may choose to eat them anyway. For example, Jason loved Chinese food. He ate it two or three times a week until he was diagnosed with Crohn's. After that, he realized that his digestive system couldn't take it. He had severe pain and diarrhea every time he ate it. For many months Jason did not eat Chinese food, as he had decided that the pain afterwards wasn't worth the pleasure of the taste going down his throat. But after a while, he missed his shrimp with lobster sauce, roast pork lo mein, spare ribs, and egg rolls so much that he decided to eat some of his favorite foods, despite the symptoms he knew it would bring. Jason still gets diarrhea from Chinese food when he eats it, so he doesn't eat it that often anymore.

On the other hand, there will be foods that you will find cause you increased physical symptoms, and you may never eat them again; it simply won't be worth it to you. How do you know what foods these are? Initially, you don't know. You will have to eat particular foods, experience increased diarrhea, and then you'll know which foods cause your symptoms to increase (sorry). There are no rules that say, "If you eat X food, Y will happen to you."

The trial and error system of figuring out the foods that are appropriate for you may be difficult because of your uncertainty of your body's response. Nobody wants to ingest food that will cause them discomfort, diarrhea, and pain. However, only your body knows how it is going to react to Chinese food, popcorn, chicken, and/or ice cream. Sometimes physicians may put you on a special diet; not because food causes Crohn's disease, but to help your body feel better through decreasing your diarrhea. Food does not cause Crohn's disease. If your disease is active, however, food may make your symptoms of diarrhea and abdominal pain worse.

Special Diets

Some physicians place people with Crohn's disease on special diets in order to minimize the symptoms that they may experience. Low-residue diets are commonly prescribed for people who have active disease. Low-residue diets entail eating foods that are bland, and are not considered roughage, such as broccoli, lettuce, vegetables, etc. It is important to note here that low-residue diets do not prevent your disease from becoming active, nor do they stop your diarrhea. Low-residue diets are diets that are "kind to your bowel," if you will. It is a specific way of eating that aids in decreasing the number of trips required to use the bathroom. Foods on low-residue diets, such as broiled chicken and baked potatoes, are easier for your digestive tract to absorb and not as irritating to your bowel as other foods, such as vegetables, peppers, and lettuce.

Example of a Low-Residue Diet

Breakfast: Toasted plain bagel (no seeds); with butter or margarine, banana, or cereal

Lunch: Turkey sandwich, no lettuce or tomatoes; pretzels, Gatorade

Dinner: Broiled chicken; baked potato OR pasta plain with butter (no sauce); parmesan cheese

The example of the low-residue diet shown above is typical of what patients who have been prescribed low-residue diets may eat. How long do you usually stay on a low-residue diet? It depends on the severity of your disease and varies from individual to individual. This is just another example of a situation where there are no hard and fast rules that apply to everyone with this disease.

If you are going to deviate from a prescribed eating regimen, remember to inform your physician so that the two of you can evaluate your disease activity as adequately as possible. Remember that deviating from a prescribed diet may not help you heal faster. Eating regimens are not the only factors affecting your digestive process. Sometimes your emotions may influence the digestive process via your eating habits, too.

Emotions and Eating Patterns

Do you ever wonder what kind of effect your feelings, or your emotions, have on your eating habits? Emotions can affect everyone's eating habits, not just those of the people with Crohn's disease. Some people, when they are emotionally upset, eat more than they usually do, and when they feel well, they don't eat much at all. Conversely, some people eat much more when they are happy, and don't eat at all when they are sad. There are those people who can easily identify when their eating habits are affected by their emotions and there are some people who do not consider that their eating habits might have been affected as a result of their feelings; indeed, they may not have been.

Your feelings may affect your eating patterns or they may not. However, as a person with Crohn's disease, increased awareness of the effect of your emotions (or lack thereof) on your eating habits can be important to you. Why? As previously stated, your nutritional health is important to your overall health. If your eating habits are influenced by your emotions, that may have an impact on your nutritional status. Your disease process and/or your medications may influence your emotions, as well, which, in turn, may indirectly affect your eating habits.

Also, if you recognize that your emotions are at the root of any change in your eating patterns, you can take action to make yourself feel better and to rectify the situation and prevent nutritional difficulties from arising while improving your nutritional status. The emotions of denial, depression, and anxiety have been discussed in other parts of this book. Now let's look at these feelings in the context of your eating habits.

Denial

If you are in denial, you may never have thought about how your eating habits may be influenced by your feelings. Perhaps your feelings don't influence your eating patterns. Regardless of whether or not you say you're sick, and despite the activity (or lack thereof) of disease in your body, your feelings may influence the types and amounts of food you eat, as well as how you digest them. The mechanisms in your body that influence this process are less important than your awareness that the process exists.

In this context, it is beneficial to you to understand how feelings can affect the eating habits of all people, regardless of whether or not they have Crohn's disease. This is particularly worthwhile for you to note, because healthy eating habits can assist you in fighting potential difficulties that might arise because of your disease process.

For instance, Samantha is a twenty-four-year-old woman who was asked to be a bridesmaid at her friend's wedding. She has Crohn's disease and was very nervous about needing to use a bathroom both prior to and during the ceremony. Consequently, the day of the wedding she made sure to eat a little bit in the morning and periodically throughout the day. Samantha knew that if she didn't eat at all she would go to the bathroom even more than if she ate a little bit several times throughout the day. She also knew that there would be a long period of time that she wouldn't eat anything at all because of the ceremony. Thus, she circumvented her need to use the bathroom by eating only at those times when she knew her body would respond in a way that would enable her to fulfill her wedding obligations and her digestive needs.

Deny, Deny, Deny

Trudy, a fifty-three-year-old woman with long-term Crohn's disease, went through many periods of denial. She would start having symptoms of diarrhea and cramping, stomach pain, bloating, and have the need to visit the rest room much more frequently. Instead of adjusting her eating patterns, sometimes she blamed the symptoms on "bad Mexican" or "stale Chinese" and continued to eat the foods that irritated her intestinal tract. Or, she blamed the symptoms (which could also include fever and lethargy) on a flu bug, or stomach virus. By the time she would finally admit that it was the Crohn's disease, she would be in a full-fledged flare-up (active disease) and would need to take medication and retreat to a very limited diet. Trudy's denial ultimately left her symptoms untreated longer than necessary. If you begin to experience physical symptoms of Crohn's disease, the kindest thing you can do for yourself is to start a food regimen that you know won't bother you. You can help yourself decrease the amount of diarrhea, etc., and perhaps even the intensity of the flare-up.

Depression

Depression may also influence your eating patterns. In fact, one of the symptoms of clinical depression is a change in appetite. Feeling sad or depressed may make you feel like not eating at all, or eating until you are too full to move. Only you know what your eating habits are like when you are sad. Either extreme can cause you difficulties. Good nutritional health will assist you in fighting the disease activity in your body; it is up to you to do everything you can to keep both your body and your mind as healthy as possible. Eating either too much or too little is not the way to maintain a well-balanced eating regimen.

As stated earlier, it is not hard to become sad or depressed when you are not feeling physically well. It is what you *do* about your feelings that makes the difference. If you know that your eating habits change when you are sad, make the effort that is required *not* to change your eating habits. You can still feel sad or depressed, but don't stop eating or start bingeing. If you are the type of person who can't eat when you are sad, try to eat a little bit many times throughout the day. If you are the type of person who eats constantly when you are sad, try to stop yourself from snacking all day. Use common sense. Don't place yourself at further risk.

You know what your eating habits are like, and when they have changed. Perhaps you pay attention to the role your emotions play in your stomach, perhaps not. Becoming aware of the influence your feelings have on your eating habits certainly can't hurt. Depending on the type of person you are, your emotions may or may not affect your physical being (e.g., increase your symptoms). When your eating habits and your emotions are out of whack, it is harder for your body to function as it does when you are feeling okay. Everyone feels sad at times. Increasing your awareness of the influence of your emotions on the rest of your body will assist you. Furthermore, depression isn't the only emotion that can influence your eating habits.

Anxiety

Anxiety, or nervous feelings, may also affect your eating habits. In fact, there are many people who don't have Crohn's disease who get an "upset stomach" when they are nervous. You don't have to have Crohn's disease to have anxiety (or feelings of any kind) affect your digestive system. Increasing your awareness of how feelings of anxiety and tension affect your eating habits helps to keep your eating well balanced during those times when you may feel both physically and emotionally compromised.

Anxiety or fear can be detrimental to both your eating habits and your psyche. As previously discussed, the best way to combat your anxiety is to identify it and take steps to alleviate your fears. In the context of your eating habits, however, this may not be easy to do. Sometimes, people become so anxious, the thought of food prevents them from being able to swallow. If you find that anxiety affects you in this manner, you might consider seeking assistance from someone who specializes in treating anxiety, to help you to overcome your specific fears. Anxiety can be paralyzing in a variety of situations if you allow it to be. When it affects your eating, it is especially important to seek outside assistance, so as not to further disrupt your physical and emotional health.

As a person with Crohn's disease, paying attention to how your emotions affect your eating habits and digestive process can be really helpful. Being aware of how your emotions affect your digestion of food can assist you in identifying ways in which to correct or modify your eating patterns. This awareness may assist you to fight the infection and/or disease process by maintaining your nutritional status, as opposed to weakening your immune system because of lack of nutrition, thus compromising your physical health further.

Medications and Eating Patterns

The medications that you take may also influence your eating patterns. Certain medications prescribed for Crohn's disease affect your entire body, not just your digestive system. Consequently, medications that you might be taking may affect both your emotional state and your appetite. Those of you who take prednisone may find that you are regularly hungry. See chapter 3 for a discussion of how different medications might influence your emotions. However, medications may also influence your eating habits.

Prednisone, for instance, is known for its effect on appetite. One possible side effect of prednisone is that it may increase or decrease your appetite. The use of prednisone results in reduction of calcium absorption, as previously discussed. It also increases the breakdown of proteins in your system. For some people, long-term use of prednisone results in increased appetite. There are many people who take prednisone who will say something like, "I just can't get the food in fast enough." The higher the dosage of prednisone and the longer you take it, the more likely you are to experience its side effects. Also, some people say they experience a decrease in appetite when they take prednisone. Remember that everyone's body is chemically different, and everyone's Crohn's disease is different. Thus, how prednisone influences you and your eating patterns might be both similar to and different from other people you know with the disease.

Mesalamine 5ASA, or drugs such as Pentasa, Asacol, and olsalazine (Dipentum), reduce folate absorption. Hence, some physicians will suggest that you take folic acid to compensate for the lack of folate absorption in your body. Folic acid aids in formation of red blood cells, and thus, helps to prevent anemia. If you are concerned about the influence of your medication(s) on your eating patterns discuss your concerns with your physician.

The longer you have Crohn's disease, the greater your capacity will be to ascertain which foods you can and cannot eat, because you will know which foods will make you feel crampy and have increased diarrhea. When you are diagnosed, it is difficult to know what you can and cannot eat, because you think everything you eat makes you sick. Sometimes, unfortunately, because of the disease process (not the food), that is the truth. Although there is no given diet or eating regimen that you can follow to prevent the disease, take some comfort in the fact that you can control what goes into your mouth. You can control what foods you eat. Only you make those decisions. There are so many different mechanisms at work in your body that you cannot control throughout the entire disease process. Take the opportunity to control what you can, to serve yourself in the healthiest manner you can.

Some Final Remarks

The remainder of this book provides you with bibliographical references and additional resources where you can obtain information about your disease. Access these informational sources or not, that's up to you. It may not be pleasant to hear (or read) about the consequences of Crohn's disease, especially if you've not been really sick. If you have been really sick, you have information from the University of Life Experiences that may be of assistance to others. The more people who know about this disease and its possible ramifications, the easier it will be for people with Crohn's disease to live with it.

Hopefully, you have found some of the information in these pages helpful. If you do not take anything else from this book, please remember that (1) perception is everything and (2) you are not your disease. One day there will be a cure for this disease. Until that time, try to make the most of every moment of your life—whether you are sick or not. Appreciate the caring and wonderful people around you. For it is my belief that *people matter*. It is the people who are a part of your life who truly give it meaning: illness is simply a small component of your whole life.

Appendix A

Glossary of Terms

Abscess: an internal collection of pus; infected area.

Alternative treatments: treatments not empirically based in Western medicine.

Anastomosis: the process of sewing the ends of intestine together.

Anemic: iron-deficient; decreased amounts of hemoglobin in red blood cells.

Arthralgia: pains in the joints.

Ciproflaxin (Cipro): antibiotic used to treat Crohn's disease.

Colectomy: surgical removal of the colon.

Colitis: inflammation of the colon, or large intestine.

Comorbid condition: more than one condition or illness that is present in the body.

Continent ileostomy: Kock pouch; the surgical creation of an ileal pouch inside the abdomen to collect waste after colectomy for people with ulcerative colitis; usually performed on people who've had a permanent ileostomy, but who don't wish to wear an external pouch, or bag. Not indicated for people who have Crohn's disease.

Crohn's colitis: Crohn's disease that is located in the colon, or large intestine.

Erethyma nodosm: red lumps on the legs; an extra-intestinal manifestation of Crohn's disease.

Fissures: cuts (usually in the area of the anus).

Fistulas: an abnormal opening between two loops of intestine, or between the intestine and another structure such as the bladder or skin. Symptom of Crohn's disease. There are different types: **Internal fistula:** an abnormal opening in the intestine that leads to another part of the body. **Perianal fistulas** are external tracts that may form from one area of the rectum to another.

Folic acid: one of the vitamins that helps to maintain red blood cells.

Gut: another word for bowel or intestine.

Ileoanal anastomosis: operation used for people who have ulcerative colitis. After a colectomy, an internal pouch is made from the ileum and attached above the anus. Also known as "pull through" or Park's operation.

Ileostomy: surgical procedure that allows waste to pass into a pouch outside the body.

Maintenance medication: any type of medication that the doctor prescribes, even when the Crohn's patient is feeling well, to keep the patient asymptomatic.

Ostomy: the surgically formed opening that serves as the exit site for connections the surgeon makes from the bowel or intestine to the outside of the body.

Perianal: area around the anal opening.

Phlegmon: suppurative swelling.

Proctocolectomy: an operation that removes the entire colon and rectum.

Pyoderma gangrenosm: skin rashes; one of the extra-intestinal manifestations of Crohn's disease.

Remission: a decrease in physical symptoms and return to good health.

Resection: a type of operation that removes, or cuts the diseased portion of intestine out of the body; the remaining two ends of the intestines are then tied back together by the surgeon; the reattachment is called *anastomosis* (see above).

Skin tags: new growths of tissue around the anal area.

Stoma: an opening from the abdomen from which waste can pass. It is located outside of the body, created from the end of the intestine, and sewn into the wall of the abdomen.

Stricture: narrowed portion of the intestine.

Suture: stitches.

Tenesmus: the feeling of urgency that causes you to seek a rest room.

Tolerance: when the efficacy of a drug decreases because the body has grown to tolerate it and needs more of the drug to take effect.

Ulcerative colitis: another type of inflammatory bowel disease. Ulcerative colitis affects only the colon.

Uveitis: eye inflammation; an extra-intestinal manifestation of Crohn's disease.

Appendix B

Additional Resources

American College of Gastroenterology
4900 B South 31st Street
Arlington, VA 22206-1656
(800) 978-7666
http://www.acg.gi.org

American Gastroenterology Association (AGA)
7910 Woodmont Avenue, 7th Floor
Bethesda, MD 20814
(301) 654-2055
http://www.gastro.org

American Medical Association (AMA)
515 North State Street
Chicago, IL 60610
(312) 464-5000
http://ww.ama-assn.org

American Society for Parenteral and Enteral Nutrition (ASPEN)
8630 Fenton Street, Suite 412
Silver Spring, MD 20910
(301) 587-6315
(800) 727-4567
http://www.clinnutr.org

The Crohn's and Colitis Foundation of America, Inc. (CCFA)
National Headquarters
386 Park Avenue South, 17th Floor
New York, NY 10016-8804
(800) 932-2423
http://ww.ccfa.org

National Institute of Diabetes and Digestion and Kidney Diseases
   (NIDDK)
9000 Rockville Pike
Bethesda, MD 20894
(301) 496-3583
http://www.nim.nih.gov

United Ostomy Association, Inc. (UOA)
19772 MacArthur, Suite 200
Irvine, CA 92612-2405
(800) 826-0826
http://www.uoa.org

References

Adler, D. 1992. Pregnancy, fertility, and contraception in inflammatory bowel disease. In *Management of Inflammatory Bowel Disease*, edited by Burton I. Korelitz and Norman Sohn. New York: Mosby Yearbook.

Alic, M. 2000. Crohn's disease epidemiology at the turn of the century. *American Journal of Gastroenterology* 95(1):321-323.

Andres, P. G., and L. S. Friedmann. 1999. The Crohn's and colitis knowledge score: A test for measuring patient knowledge in inflammatory bowel disease. *Gastroenterology Clinics of North America* 28(2):255-281.

Antoni, M. H., and N. Schneiderman. 1998. HIV/AIDS. In *Comprehensive Clinical Psychology*, edited by A. Bellack and M. Hersen. New York: Elsevier Science.

Antoni, M. H., N. Schneiderman, and G. Ironson. 2000. Stress management for HIV infection. *Society of Behavioral Medicine Clinical Research Guidebook Series*. New Jersey: Erlbaum Press.

Baird, D. D., M. Narendranathan, and R. S. Sandler. 1990. Increased risk of preterm birth for women with inflammatory bowel disease. *Gastroenterology* 99(4):987-994.

Bambrick, M., V. W. Fazio, T. L. Hull, and G. Pucel. 1996. Sexual function following restorative proctocolectomy in women. *Diseases of the Colon and Rectum* 39(6):610-614.

Basson, R. 1998. Sexual health of women with disabilities. *Canadian Medical Association Journal* 159(4):359-362.

Botoman, V. A., G. F. Bonner, D. and A. Botoman. 1998. Management of inflammatory bowel disease. *American Family Physician* 57(1): 57-68.

Burakoff, R. 1993.Questions and answers about pregnancy and IBD. In *IBD File* edited by CCFA, Inc. New York: CCFA, Inc..

———. 1995. Fertility and pregnancy in inflammatory bowel disease. In *Inflammatory Bowel Disease*, 4th ed., edited by J. B. Kirsner and R. G. Shorter. Baltimore: Williamson & Wilkins.

Casselith, B. R., E. J. Lusk, T. B. Strouse, D. S. Miller, L. L. Brown, P. A. Cross, et al. 1984. Psychosocial status in chronic illness. *New England Journal of Medicine* 311(8):506-509.

Chapman, C. R. 1978. Pain: The perceptions of noxious events. In *The Psychology of Pain,* edited by R. A. Sternbach. New York: Lippincott-Raven Publishers.

Crohn's and Colitis Foundation of America (CCFA). 2000. Brochure. New York: CCFA.

Damgaard, B., A. Wettergren, and P. Kirkegaard. 1995. Social and sexual function following ileal pouch-anal anastomosis. *Diseases of the Colon and Rectum* 38(3):286-89.

Drossman, D. A. 1995. Psychosocial factors in ulcerative colitis and Crohn's disease. In *Inflammatory Bowel Disease*, 4th ed., edited by J. B. Kirsner and R. G. Shorter. Baltimore: Williamson & Wilkins.

———. 1996. Inflammatory bowel disease. In *Quality of Life and Pharmacoeconomics in Clinical Trials,* edited by B. Spilker. Philadelphia: Lippincott-Raven Publishers.

Duffy, L. C., M. A. Zielenzy, J. R. Marshall, T. E. Byers, M. M. Weiser, J. F. Phillips, et al. 1991. Relevance of major stress events as an indicator of disease activity prevalence in inflammatory bowel disease. *Behavioral Medicine* 17(3):101-110.

Eysselein, V. E. 2000. Reduction of stress: A new therapeutic goal in the treatment of inflammatory bowel disease. *Inflammatory Bowel Diseases* 6(2):153-154.

Fullwood, A., and D. A. Drossman. 1995. The relationship of psychiatric illness with gastrointestinal disease. *Annual Review of Medicine* 46:483-496.

Garrett, J. W., and D. A Drossman. 1990. Health status in inflammatory bowel disease: Biological and behavioral considerations. *Gastroenterology* 99(1):90-96.

Garrett, V. D., P. J. Brantley, G. N. Jones, and G. T. McKnight. 1991. The relation between daily stress and Crohn's disease. *Journal of Behavioral Medicine* 14(1):87-96.

Gerson L. B., and G. Triadafilopoulos. 2000. Palliative care in inflammatory bowel disease. *Inflammatory Bowel Diseases* 6(3):228-243.

Gloeckner, M. 1983. Partner reaction following ostomy surgery. *Journal of Sex and Marital Therapy* 9(3):182-190.

Greene, B. R., E. B. Blanchard, and C. K. Wan. 1994. Long-term monitoring of psychosocial stress and symptomatology in inflammatory bowel disease. *Behavior, Research, and Therapy* 32(2):217-226.

Greenwood, Jan. 1992. *The IBD Nutrition Book.* New York: John Wiley & Sons.

Heller, A. D. 1992. Nutrition in patients with inflammatory bowel disease. In *Management of Inflammatory Bowel Disease,* edited by B. I. Korelitz and N. Sohn. St. Louis: Mosby Yearbook.

Huish M., D. Kumar, and C. Stones. 1998. Stoma surgery and sexual problems in ostomates. *Sexual and Marital Therapy* 13(3):311-324.

James, D. 1993. Questions and answers about gynecological issues and IBD. In *IBD File,* edited by CCFA, Inc. New York: CCFA, Inc..

Janowitz, H. D. 1994. Assessing the patient's clinical status and the degree of impairment. In *Inflammatory Bowel Disease: A Clinical Approach,* edited by H. D. Janowitz. Oxford, England: Oxford University Press (original work published 1985).

Kane, S. 1999. Women's issues in inflammatory bowel disease. In *IBD File,* edited by CCFA, Inc. New York: CCFA, Inc.

Keefe, F. J., and J. D. Beckham. 1994. Behavioral medicine. In *Cognitive and Behavioral Interventions: An Empirical Approach to Mental Health Problems,* edited by L. W. Craighead, W. E. Craighead, A. E. Kazdin, and M. J. Mahoney. Boston: Allyn and Bacon.

Korelitz, B. I. 1998. Inflammatory bowel disease and pregnancy. *Gastroenterology Clinics of North America* 27(1):213-224.

McCaul, K. D., and J. M. Malott. 1984. Distraction and coping with pain. *Psychological Bulletin* 95:516-533.

McLeod, R. 1997. The pelvic pouch procedure remains an excellent option for most patients with ulcerative colitis requiring surgery. In *Inflammatory Bowel Diseases,* edited by P. Banks and D. Present. New York: CCFA, Inc., 3(3):236-238.

McKegney, F. P., R. D. Gordon, and S. M. Levine. 1970. A psychosomatic comparison of patients with ulcerative colitis and Crohn's disease. *Psychosomatic Medicine* 32:153-166.

Metcalf, A. M., R. R. Dozios, and K. A. Kelly. 1986. Sexual function in women after proctocolectomy. *Annals of Surgery* 204(6): 624-627.

Monk, M., A. I. Medeloff, C. I. Siegel, and A. Lilienfeld. 1970. An epidemiological study of ulcerative colitis and regional enteritis among adults in Baltimore. *Journal of Chronic Disease* 22: 565-578.

Moser, M. A. J., N. B. Okun, D. C. Mayes, and R. J. Bailey. 2000. Crohn's disease, pregnancy, and birth weight. *American Journal of Gastroenterology* 95(4):1021-1026.

North, C. S., D. H. Alpers, J. E. Helzer, E. L. Spitznagel, and R. E. Clouse. 1991. Do life events or depression exacerbate inflammatory bowel disease? A prospective study. *Annals of Internal Medicine* 114(5):381-386.

Olbrisch, M. E., and S. W. Ziegler. 1982. Psychological adjustment to inflammatory bowel disease: Informational control and private self-consciousness. *Journal of Chronic Diseases* 35:573-580.

O'Keefe, S. J. D., and B. G. Rossner. 1994. Nutrition and inflammatory bowel disease. In *Inflammatory Bowel Disease: From Bench to Bedside,* edited by S. R. Targan and F. Shanahan. Baltimore: Williams & Wilkins.

O'Sullivan M. O., and C. O'Morain. 2000. Patient knowledge in inflammatory bowel disease. *American Journal of Gastroenterology* 95(8):2128-2129.

Peppercorn, M. A. 1999. Medical therapy. In *Inflammatory Bowel Disease: A Guide for Patients and their Families,* edited by S. H. Stein and R. P. Rood. Philadelphia: Lippincott-Raven Publishers.

Ramchandani, D., B. Schindler, and J. Katz. 1994. Evolving concepts of psychopathology in inflammatory bowel disease. *Medical Clinics of North America* 78(6):1321-1330.

Richardson, J. H., , J. W. Present, and M. Merrick. 1999. Making a difference: The role of CCFA and its support of patients. In *Inflammatory Bowel Disease: A Guide for Patients and their Families,* edited by S. H. Stein and T. P. Rood. Philadelphia: Lippincott-Raven Publishers.

Robertson, D. A., J. Jay, I. Diamond, and J. G. Edwards. 1989. Personality profile and affective state of patients with inflammatory bowel disease. *Gut* 30 (5):623-626.

Rogers, A. I. 2000. Paper presented to the Division of Gastroenterology, University of Miami School of Medicine. December. Paper presentation.

Rolandelli, R. H. 1994. Surgical treatment of Crohn's disease. In *Inflammatory Bowel Disease: From Bench to Bedside,* edited by S. R. Targan and F. Shanahan. Baltimore: Williams & Wilkins.

Sachar D. B. 1997. Inflammatory bowel disease. Paper presented at the meeting of the American College of Gastroenterology Post-Graduate Course, Chicago, Illinois. October.

Sandler, R. S. 1994. Epidemiology of inflammatory bowel disease. In *Inflammatory Bowel Disease: From Bench to Bedside,* edited by S. R. Targan and F. Shanahan. Baltimore: Williams & Wilkins.

Saubermann, L. J., and J. L. Wolf. 1999. Inflammatory bowel disease and pregnancy. In *Inflammatory Bowel Disease: A Guide for Patients and Their Families,* edited by S. H. Stein and R. P. Rood. New York: CCFA, Inc.

Scaglia, M., E. Bronsino., V. Canino, et al. 1993.The impact of conventional proctocolectomy on sexual function. *Minerva Chirurgia* 48(17):903-910.

Scaglia, M., G. G. Delaini, and L. Hulten. 1992. Sexual dysfunctions after conventional proctocolectomy. *Chirurgia Italiana* 44(5-6): 230-242.

Schwarz, S. P., and E. B. Blanchard. 1990. Inflammatory bowel disease: A review of the psychological assessment and treatment literature. *Annals of Behavioral Medicine* 12(3):95-105.

————. 1991. Evaluation of a psychological treatment for inflammatory bowel disease. *Behavior Research and Therapy* 29(2):167-177.

Seidel, S. A., S. E. Peach, M. Newman, and K. W. Sharp. 1999. Ileoanal pouch procedures: Clinical outcomes and quality of life assessment. *American Surgeon* 65(1):40-46.

Sessions, J. T., D. Raft, and S. Tate. 1978. The severity of Crohn's disease does not correlate with life stress, depression and anxiety. *Gastroenterology* 74(5):1144.

Tiainen, J., M. Matikainen, and K. M. Hiltunen. 1999. Ileal J-pouch: Anal anastomosis, sexual dysfunction, and fertility. *Scandinavian Journal of Gastroenterology* 34(2):185-188.

Talal, A. H., and D. A. Drossman. 1995. Psychosocial factors in inflammatory bowel disease. *Gastroenterology Clinics of North America* 24(3):699-716.

Trachter, A. B., A. H. Sellers, A. Katell, and M. Ishii. 2000. The effects of psychological symptoms and personality traits on disease activation among inflammatory bowel disease patients. Dissertation. See www.cps.nova.edu (dissertation is not online).

Amy Trachter, Psy.D., Ph.D., is a clinical psychologist specializing in the treatment of medical patients, and a researcher whose interests focus on the Inflammatory Bowel Diseases. Dr. Trachter has been facilitating support groups for the Crohn's and Colitis Foundation of America (CCFA) for over a decade, currently serves on the board of directors for the South Florida chapter of CCFA, and is a member of the organization's National Patient Education Committee.

Some Other
New Harbinger Titles

The Trigger Point Therapy Workbook, Item TPTW $19.95

Fibromyalgia and Chronic Myofascial Pain Syndrome, Item FMS $19.95

Kill the Craving, Item KC $18.95

Rosacea, Item ROSA $13.95

Thinking Pregnant, Item TKPG $13.95

Shy Bladder Syndrome, Item SBDS $13.95

Help for Hairpullers, Item HFHP $13.95

Coping with Chronic Fatigue Syndrome, Item CFS $13.95

The Stop Smoking Workbook, Item SMOK $17.95

Multiple Chemical Sensitivity, Item MCS $16.95

Breaking the Bonds of Irritable Bowel Syndrome, Item IBS $14.95

Parkinson's Disease and the Art of Moving, Item PARK $15.95

The Addiction Workbook, Item AWB $17.95

The Interstitial Cystitis Survival Guide, Item ICS $14.95

Illness and the Art of Creative Self-Expression, Item EXPR $13.95

Don't Leave it to Chance, Item GMBL $13.95

The Chronic Pain Control Workbook, 2nd edition, Item PN2 $18.95

Perimenopause, 2nd edition, Item PER2 $16.95

The Family Recovery Guide, Item FAMG $15.95

Healthy Baby, Toxic World, Item BABY $15.95

I'll Take Care of You, Item CARE $12.95

Call **toll free, 1-800-748-6273,** or log on to our online bookstore at **www.newharbinger.com** to order. Have your Visa or Mastercard number ready. Or send a check for the titles you want to New Harbinger Publications, Inc., 5674 Shattuck Ave., Oakland, CA 94609. Include $4.50 for the first book and 75¢ for each additional book, to cover shipping and handling. (California residents please include appropriate sales tax.) Allow two to five weeks for delivery.

Prices subject to change without notice.